Contents

Foreword

To have ten doctors newly trained in their vocation produce a *Guide to General Practice* is an exciting event. Here are clearly perceived needs met by a joint effort whilst still in training. Here is courage to help constructively those in the same position. Here is a demonstration of realistic self help.

This collection of data for every day represents an essential minimum for the doctor in his first plunge into General Practice. It gives information often buried in the experience of their elders or in books and circulars.

Such a guide should be a useful cornerstone on which to build. It should be followed by many editions as experience gained by the contributors is strengthened by increasing confidence.

These ten authors in training have set a high example that bodes well for the future of General Practice.

E. V. Kuenssberg
President of the Royal College of
General Practitioners

Preface to third edition

The *Guide* has stood the test of twelve years everyday use on the doctor's desk or in the black bag. This, the third edition, revises and updates the original work and incorporates changes brought about by the 1990 Contract. To extend the book's usefulness for ready reference, we have incorporated a section on emergency care in general practice which is based on the chapter on emergencies by Simon Street and Ken Burch in *Essential Primary Care* (Blackwell Scientific Publications 1987).

Andrew Wilkinson   June 1990
Simon Street
Mike McGhee

Preface to first edition

This handbook was written by general practice trainees during their training year. It is intended for trainees but should be of value to locums, assistants and new partners. It is a guide to the management of problems commonly encountered by doctors new to general practice. Details of medical treatment have been avoided deliberately. The material was selected from our experiences during the year. We were assisted by our trainers and other doctors to whom we are most grateful. We are also grateful to Jackie Sumner for her secretarial work.

Martyn Agass   Richard Lloyd   August 1978
Jeremy Bray   Michael McGhee
Robert Cave   Simon Street
Gillian Dean   Keith Sumner
Shirley Elliott   Andrew Wilkinson

The black bag

BLACK BAG — DIAGNOSTIC

Adhesive plasters
Clinical thermometer
Fluoresceine sticks
Foetal stethoscope
Gloves, jelly and tissues
Low reading thermometer
Needles
Ophthalmoscope
Otoscope
Patella hammer
Peak flow meter
Sharps box
Sphygmomanometer
Stethoscope
Swabs and specimen containers and transport medium
Syringes
Tape measure
Tongue depressors
Torch
Tourniquet
Tuning fork
Urine and blood dip sticks
Vaginal speculum

BLACK BAG – THERAPEUTIC

Injectable drugs
Adrenaline
Antiarrhythmics
Antibiotic
Anticonvulsant
Antiemetic
Antihistamine
Bronchodilator
Corticosteroid
Diuretic
Ergometrine
Glucagon or IV Dextrose
Major and minor tranquilliser
Opiate analgesic
Opiate antagonist

Oral drugs
Antacid
Antibiotics
Antidiarrhoeal
Antihistamine
Aspirin
Bronchodilator
Corticosteroid
Diuretic
Major and minor analgesic
Sedative
Sugar lumps

Miscellaneous
Bronchodilator for nebuliser
Eyedrops
Glycerol suppositories
Ipecaccuanha
Paediatric antibiotics
Paediatric paracetamol
Trinitrin

Drugs given from bag should be in a suitable container—glass or plastic, labelled with the following:

Patient's name
Drug name, dosage and quantity
Instructions, warnings and precautions
Name and address of Doctor
Date
Warning: 'Keep out of reach of children'

BLACK BAG – ADMINISTRATIVE

Coins for telephone or phone card
Continuation cards
Controlled drugs record book
Dispensing forms
Emergency Treatment forms
Envelopes
Headed notepaper
Immediate Necessary Treatment forms
List of Chemists to dispense 'Urgent' prescriptions
Map
National Insurance Certificates
Obstetric calculator
Pathology forms
Prescription pad
Private certificates
Registration forms
Telephone numbers list
Temporary Resident forms
Therapeutic handbook

BLACK BAG – OPTIONAL EQUIPMENT

Airway
Antiseptic concentrate
Bandage and dressings
Drainage bag
ECG
Epistaxis balloon
Giving set and fluids
IV Cannula
Monitor/defibrillator

Nebuliser
Peak flow meter
Oxygen/ventilator
Scissors
Sterile dressing pack
Steristrips
Suturing equipment
Urinary catheters, bags and spigots

BLACK BAG – OBSTETRIC

Equipment

Adult and neonatal
   endotracheal tube
Apron
Artery forceps
Calibrated jug
Dissecting forceps
Endotracheal tube
Episiotomy scissors
Giving set and fluids
IV cannula
Gloves
Laryngoscope
Light source
Mucus extractor

Needle holder
Neonatal laryngoscope
Obstetric cream
Obstetric forceps
Perineal retractor
Pudendal block needle
Sample bottles
Space blanket
Sterile dressing sheets
Suturing equipment
Swabs
Syringes and needles
Umbilical clamps
Urinary catheter

Drugs

Antibiotic
Concentrated antiseptic
Diazepam
Ergometrine
Hydrallazine/Nifedepine

Local anaesthetic
Pethidine
Syntometrine
Vitamin K_1
Opiate antagonist

BLACK BAG – ROAD TRAFFIC ACCIDENT

Minimal equipment
Airway
Field dressings
Fire extinguisher
Fluorescent jacket
Giving set and fluid
Gloves
IV cannula
Reflective warning triangle
Torch
Triage labels and waterproof pen
Triangular bandages

Additional equipment
Blankets
Camera (with flash)
Cardiac monitor and defibrillator
Chest drain
Cut-down and surgical set
Dictaphone or notebook
Drugs for resuscitation
Endotracheal tubes
Entonox
Equipment for manual ventilation
Equipment for examination and blood samples
First aid kit including field and burns dressings
Flutter valve
Inflatable splints
Laryngoscope
Oxygen
Oxymeter
Protective and identifying clothing
Radio telephone
Sharps box
Sucker
Suturing equipment
Warning signs and flashing beacon for car

BLACK BAG – DISPENSING

Carry prepacked containers of standard amounts, labelled except for name and date dispensed.

Mark expiry date.

Mark filling level on bottles of dry powder for medicines.

Arrange collection/delivery of drugs not available from bag.

Special arrangements for drugs needing storage—vaccines, insulin.

Analgesic–mild
       –moderate
       –opioid
Antacid
Antibiotic–broad spectrum
       –metranidazole
       –penicillinase resistant
Anticoagulant
Anticonvulsant
Antidepressant
Antidiarrhoeal
Antiemetic
Antihistamine
Antiparkinsonian drug
Antispasmodic
Antipsychotic/major tranquilizers
Benzodiazepine
β blocker
Bronchodilator
Digoxin
Diuretic–K^+ supplement
      –mild
      –strong
Ear/eye preparations–antibiotic
              –steroid

BLACK BAG — DISPENSING — continued

Trinitrate
H_2 antagonist
Hypotensive
Inhalers–steroid
      –bronchodilator
Iron preparation
Laxative
Migraine preparation
NSAID
Oral contraceptives
Oral hypoglycaemic
Paediatric–antibiotic
      –antiemetic
      –antihistamine/sedative
      –electrolyte sachets
Skin–steroid
   –fungicide
Steroid

Medical practice

DESIRABLE WEIGHT CHART

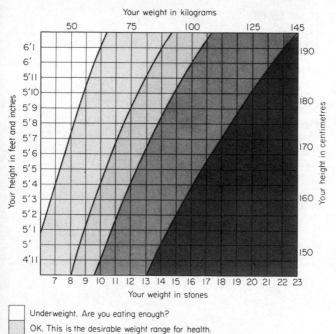

Your weight in kilograms

Your height in feet and inches

Your height in centimetres

Your weight in stones

☐ Underweight. Are you eating enough?

▨ OK. This is the desirable weight range for health.

▧ Overweight. Not likely to have much effect on your health but don't get any fatter!

▦ Fat. Your health could suffer if you don't lose weight.

■ Very fat. This is severe and treatment is urgently required.

Reproduced with the permission of Churchill Livingstone from *Treat Obesity seriously* by J. S. Garrow (1981).

DERMATOME CHART

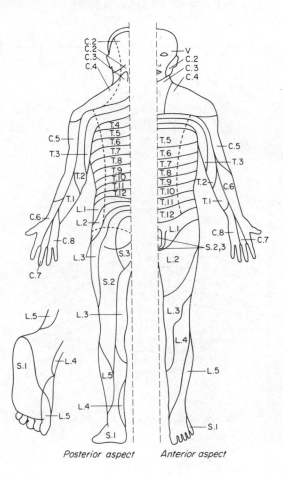

Posterior aspect   *Anterior aspect*

Reproduced with the permission of the Oxford University Press from *Brain's Clinical Neurology*, edited by R. Bannister (1978).

NORMAL VALUES OF PEAK EXPIRATORY FLOW–ADULT

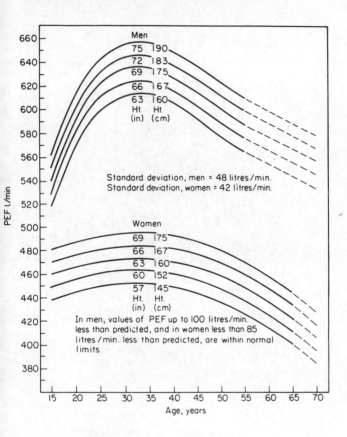

Courtesy of Clement Clarke International Ltd, Wigmore Street, London W1H 9LA

NORMAL VALUES OF PEAK
EXPIRATORY FLOW–CHILDREN

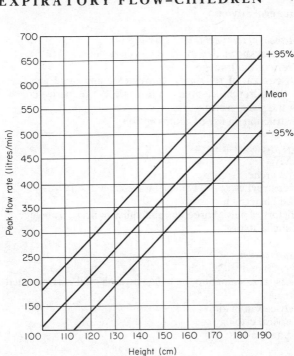

Normogram redrawn from original data of Godfrey *et al. British Journal of Diseases of the Chest*, **64**, 15 (1970). Reproduced by permission of Clement Clarke International Ltd, Wigmore Street, London W1H 9LA

11

FAMILY PLANNING

General advice

Methods of contraception
General knowledge of sex and sex function
Previous contraception
Discussion of reliability, convenience and disadvantages of
    the different methods with regard to age, parity, consort,
    and social factors
Instruction on use of contraceptives

Gynaecological history
LMP
Menarche
Menstrual cycle – frequency and complications
Past obstetric history
History of pelvic infection, abdominal or pelvic pathology
Rubella status

Examination
Weight and BP
General examination, including psychological—as indicated
Breasts
Pelvic examination
Cervical cytology
Urine analysis

Documentation
FP1001—Registration
FP1002—IUCD
FP1003—Temporary Resident

FAMILY PLANNING

The combined pill

Absolute contraindications
Thromboembolism
Severe Hypertension
Impaired Liver function
Oestrogen dependent tumours

Splenectomy
Otosclerosis
Pituitary disorder
Porphyria

Relative contraindications
More than 35 years
More than 10 years 'on the Pill'
Hypertension
Smoking
Family History of IHD
Diabetes
Depression

Migraine
Epilepsy
Renal disease
Valvular heart disease
Varicose Veins
Oligomenorrhoea
Breast Feeding
Contact Lenses

Side-effects

	Progestogen	Oestrogen
Too much	Depression	Hypertension
	Loss of libido	Recurrent migraine
	Ammenorrhoea	Premenstrual tension
	Breast discomfort	Breast discomfort
	Acne	Nausea and bloating
		Vaginal discharge
	Steady weight gain	Weight gain
Too little	Breakthrough bleeding	Breakthrough bleeding
	Menorrhagia	

Follow up
Initially 3 months

Every 6 months
Every 3 years

Weight, BP
symptom review
As above
As above plus
pelvic examination
breast examination
cervical cytology

FAMILY PLANNING

Prostogen only pill

Absolute contraindications

Thromboembolism
Severe hypertension
Impaired liver function

Splenectomy
Otosclerosis
Porphyria

Relative contraindications

Smoking
Family history of IHD
Obesity
Diabetes
Contact lenses
Previous ectopic pregnancy

Depression
Epilepsy
Renal disease
Valvular heart disease
Varicose Veins
Oligomenorrhoea

Side-effects

Too much
    Depression
    Loss of libido
    Ammennorrhoea
    Breast discomfort
    Acne
    Hirsuitism
    Steady weight gain
    Recurrent thrush
Too little
    Breakthrough bleeding
    Mennorrhagia

Follow up

Initially 3 months :
    Weight, blood pressure
    Symptom review

Every 6 months :
    As above
Every 3 years :
    As above plus—
    Pelvic examination
    Breast examination
    Cervical cytology

FAMILY PLANNING

Intra-uterine contraceptive devices

Medical history
LMP—for timing of insertion
Regularity of menses
Active infection
History of:
    Pelvic infection
    Heart valve diseases
    Anticoagulants and bleeding diatheses
    Anaemia
    Uterine malformation

Side effects
Increase in menstrual flow
Expulsion of IUCD
Lost threads
Pregnancy and ectopic pregnancy
Perforation
Infection and subsequent infertility
Pain

Follow up
After first period then annually
    Self examination
    Pelvic examination
    Side effects
    Change of IUCD – as indicated

FAMILY PLANNING

Rhythm methods
Temperature chart
Regular cycle
   'Unsafe Days' are Day 14 ± 4
Irregular cycle
   If the shortest cycle is x days and the longest cycle is y days
   then the 'safe' days are between $y-11$ and $x-18$
   Billings—Cervical mucus changes with ovulation

Barrier methods

Condom
With or without spermicidal creams or pessaries
No medical advice required

Diaphragm
Assess vaginal size and position of cervix
Follow up at 6 weeks and 6 months
Change cap every year

Traditional methods
Including coitus interruptus

Sterilisation counselling
Gynaecological or medical history
Reason for request
Stability of relationship
Attitude to parenthood
Examination
Technique of procedure
Permanence and reversibility
Low incidence of side effects or failure
Risk of recanalisation
Complications previous operation/anaesthetic

FAMILY PLANNING

Post coital contraception

Oral
Two doses of combined oral contraceptive pill at 12 hr intervals to be started not later than 72 hours after intercourse
Typically 50 mcg Ethinyloestadiol/levonorgestrel
Two tablets repeated after 12 hours

Side effects
Nausea and vomiting
Increased tubal pregnancy rate
Check that menstruation occurs within 3 weeks

IUCD
Insertion not later than 72 hours after intercourse is another effective method.
Advise subsequent contraception.

Contraception for girls under 16
The Law Lords set five 'tests' that a doctor must apply before prescribing confidentially to a girl under 16 years.
1   That the girl (although under 16 years of age) will understand the doctors advice.
2   That he/she cannot persuade her to inform her parents or to allow the doctor to inform the parents that she is seeking contraceptive advice.
3   That she is likely to begin or to continue having sexual intercourse with or without contraceptive treatment.
4   That unless she receives contraceptive advice or treatment her physical or mental health or both are likely to suffer.
5   That her best interest require the doctor to give contraceptive advice, treatment or both without the parental consent.

Doctors are advised to consult their Medical Defense organisation before prescribing contraception to girls under 16 years.

FIRST ANTENATAL VISIT

History of present pregnancy
LMP, EDD, cycle, contraception, especially OC pill

Previous obstetric history
Pregnancy, labour, puerperium
Infant (alive or stillborn), weight, sex, gestation, neonatal
    problems
Feeding

Previous gynaecological history
Abortions – spontaneous or induced
Subfertility – investigations and treatment
Pelvic and abdominal surgery

General medical history
Hypertension and cardiac disease
Tuberculosis
Diabetes
Urinary tract infection, renal disease
STD and HIV exposure
Varicose veins
Psychiatric history—previous postnatal depression

Family history
Twins
Congenital abnormalities
General medical

Social history
Marital status
Smoking
Alcohol/drugs
Accommodation

Drugs
Current therapy
Allergies
Transfusions

FIRST ANTENATAL VISIT – continued

Examination
Weight, height, shoe size
Teeth, mucous membranes
Varicose veins
Blood pressure, heart sounds
Breasts
Abdomen – fundal height
Pelvic examination, cervical smear

Investigation
Urine, for microscopy, glucose, protein culture
Hb, blood group, WR, Rh antibodies
Rubella antibodies
Hepatitis antibodies
HIV
Consider ultrasound scan

Discussion
Antenatal care, parenthood classes
Amnio-centesis and genetic counselling
Diet, smoking, alcohol, drugs, X rays
Sexual intercourse, relaxation exercises
Dental care
Delivery and feeding
Postnatal social support

Forms:
FP 24, FW 8 (booking)
DHSS payments, Mat Bl (26 weeks)

Referral letter
Include all significant findings from the above assessment

SUBSEQUENT ANTENATAL VISITS

Follow-up
Monthly until 28 weeks
Then fortnightly until 36 weeks
Then weekly until term

History
Estimated dates
Symptoms—bleeding, pain, dyspepsia, constipation
Foetal movements

Examination
Weight, urine analysis, BP
Oedema
Fundal height – dates?
Lie and position
Presentation
Engagement
Foetal heart

Investigations

12 weeks	Hb, antibodies
16–19 weeks	Alpha Feto Protein
28 weeks	Hb, antibodies if Rh negative
34 weeks	Hb, antibodies if Rh negative, vaginal examination and pelvic assessment

ANTENATAL CLASSES

Mothers' health
Exercise and relaxation
Diet, smoking, alcohol and pills
Mothers' questions and anxieties
Social contacts for new mothers
Maternity benefits

Hospital visit

The delivery
First, second and third stages
Pain relief
Caesarians, forceps and episiotomy
The neonate

Parentcraft
Feeding
Clothing
Bathing
Playing
Toys and equipment
Fathers' role
Emotional demands

FINAL POSTNATAL VISIT

Delivery
Date of delivery
Mode
Sex
Birth weight
Antenatal, perinatal or postnatal complications

Infant
Mode of feeding
Weight gain

Mother
Anaemia – oral iron therapy
Breast care
Bowels
Micturition
Lochia
Menstruation
Depression

Examination
Weight and blood pressure
Anaemia
Breasts
Abdomen – size of uterus
Perineum – episiotomy, muscle tone
Vulva and vagina
Cervix
Bimanual examination of uterus
Urine
Cervical smear

Discussion
Contraception – if not already using a method
Mother – child bonding
Complete FP24 etc
Register infant in practice
Immunisation and child care
Child health surveillance form (FP/CHS)

CHILD HEALTH CLINIC

With the new contract these are being run increasingly by Health Visitors with General Practitioners.

They provide a meeting place for mothers to discuss all aspects of child health amongst themselves or with professionals.

Arrangements may vary but the doctor is usually responsible for developmental screening and is available for referrals from the health visitor. The doctor or a nurse carries out the immunisations.

Most local authorities have a planned screening programme which should be regarded as a minimum. In a typical programme a child is seen at 2 months, 8 months and 18 months.

SCHOOL CLINIC

Organised by the Specialist in Community Medicine and Child Health responsible for area school health services.

Each child should attend the clinic during his second term, with his mother, child health clinic notes and teacher's notes.

Assessment is made of emotional, intellectual, social and physical development.

Examination
Appearance, height and weight
Gait
Motor ability
Speech
Visual acuity, squints
Colour vision
Hearing, audiometry

Failure or low attainment may merit reassessment or referral to a specialist agency via the general practitioner.

CHILD ASSESSMENT

Six week check

Average baby at 6 weeks	Smiles Eyes fixate and follow past midline Quietens to sound Head level momentarily in ventral suspension
Examination	Posture prone and ventral Weight Head circumference Heart sounds and femoral pulses Genitalia and hips Eye movements and squint Palate and fontanelle
Referral	Dislocated hips Heart murmurs Cataracts Persistent primitive reflexes Abnormal tone

CHILD ASSESSMENT

Eight month check

Average baby at 8 months	Sits unsupported Thumb/finger grasp Feeds himself Responds to more than 4 sounds
Examination	Weight Head circumference Hearing Vision distant and squint Dexterity Posture and tone Heart, hips, genitalia
Referral	Heart murmurs Failure to achieve milestones Failure to thrive

CHILD ASSESSMENT

Eighteen month check

Average toddler at 18 months	Walks, runs, climbs a chair
	Three words apart from 'mama' and 'dada'
	Builds tower of 3 bricks
	Drinks from cup
Examination	General physical
	Height, weight,
	Head circumference
	Genitalia
	Heart sounds
	Ears
	Vision, squint
Referral	Failure to achieve milestones
	Non walking
	Primitive reflexes or tone

CHILD ASSESSMENT

Three year check

Average child at 3 years	Jumps down steps, stands on one leg, rides a trike
	Good language development
	Can draw a man, copy circle
	Normal socialisation with adults and other children
Examination	Height weight
	Head circumference
	General physical
	Vision and squint
	Hearing and ears
Referral	Abnormalities of above

DENVER DEVELOPMENTAL SCREENING TEST

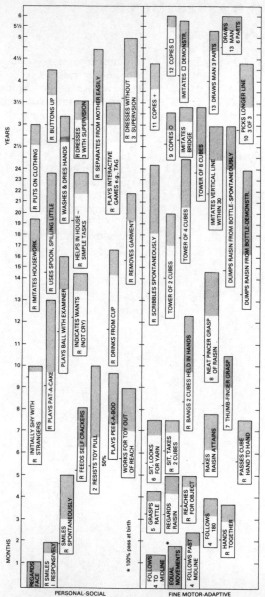

DENVER DEVELOPMENTAL
SCREENING TEST—continued

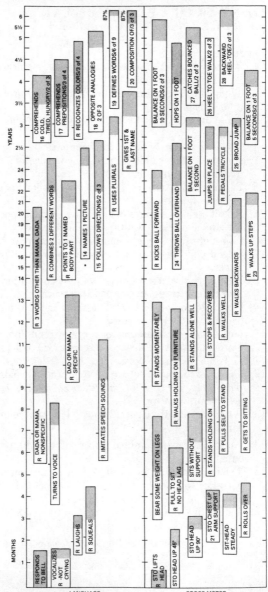

DENVER DEVELOPMENTAL
SCREENING TEST—continued

Directions

1. Try to get child to smile by smiling, talking or waving to him. Do not touch him.
2. When child is playing with toy, pull it away from him. Pass if he resists.
3. Child does not have to be able to tie shoes or button in the back.
4. Move yarn slowly in an arc from one side to the other, about 6'' above child's face. Pass if eyes follow 90° to midline. (Past midline; 180°.)
5. Pass if child grasps rattle when it is touched to the backs or tips of fingers.
6. Pass if child continues to look where yarn disappeared or tries to see where it went. Yarn should be dropped quickly from sight from tester's hand without arm movement.
7. Pass if child picks up raisin with any part of thumb and finger.
8. Pass if child picks up raisin with the ends of thumb and index finger using an overhand approach.
9. Get child to copy a circle. Pass any enclosed form. Fail continuous round motions.
10. Get child to indicate the longer of two lines (not bigger). Turn paper upside down and repeat. (3/3 or 5/6.)
11. Get child to copy a cross. Pass any crossing lines.
12. Get child to copy a square. Demonstrate if he fails.
When giving items, 9, 11 and 12, do not name the forms. Do not demonstrate 9 and 11.
13. When scoring, each pair (2 arms, 2 legs, etc.) count as one part.
14. Get child to name animal picture. (No credit for sounds only.)
15. Tell child to: Give block to Mommie; put block on table; put block on floor. Pass 2 of 3. (Do not help child by pointing, moving head or eyes.)
16. Ask child: What do you do when you are cold? . . . hungry? . . . tired? Pass 2 of 3.

DENVER DEVELOPMENTAL SCREENING TEST—continued

Directions—continued

17. Tell child to: Put block *on* table; *under* table; *in front* of chair, *behind* chair. Pass 3 of 4. (Do not help child by pointing, moving head or eyes.)
18. Ask child: If fire is hot, ice is   ?; Mother is a woman, Dad is a   ?; a horse is big, a mouse is   ?. Pass 2 of 3.
19. Ask child: What is a ball? ... lake? ... desk? ... house? ... banana? ... curtain? ... ceiling? ... hedge? ... pavement? Pass if defined in terms of use, shape, what it is made of or general category (such as banana is fruit, not just yellow). Pass 6 of 9.
20. Ask child: What is a spoon made of? ... a shoe made of? ... a door made of? (No other objects may be substituted.) Pass 3 of 3.
21. When placed on stomach, child lifts chest off table with support of forearms and/or hands.
22. When child is on back, grasp his hands and pull him to sitting. Pass if head does not hang back.
23. Child may use wall or rail only, not person. May not crawl.
24. Child must throw overhand 3 feet to within arm's reach of tester.
25. Child must perform standing broad jump over width of test sheet. (8½ inches)
26. Tell child to walk forward, heel to toe, heel within 1 inch of toe. Tester may demonstrate. Child must walk 4 consecutive steps, 2 out of 3 trials.
27. Bounce ball to child who should stand 3 feet away from tester. Child must catch ball with hands, not arms, 2 out of 3 trials.
28. Tell child to walk backward, toe to heel, toe within 1 inch of heel. Tester may demonstrate. Child must walk 4 consecutive steps, 2 out of 3 trials.

Date and behavioural observations (how child feels at time of test, relations to tester, attention span, verbal behaviour, self-confidence, etc,):

31

BOYS' HEIGHT

Longitudinal standards for weight attained at given age. The shaded areas represent the 97th and 3rd centile limits of cross-sectionally derived standards.

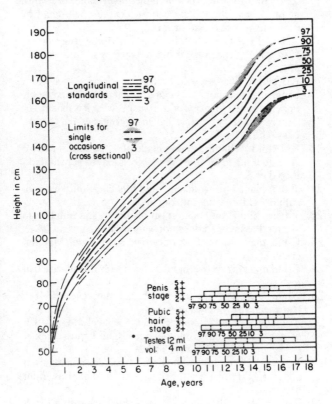

Prepared by Professor J.M. Tanner and Mr R.H. Whitehouse and reproduced by permission of Castlemead Publications, Hertford.

BOYS' WEIGHT

Longitudinal standards for weight attained at given age. The shaded areas represent the 97th and 3rd centile limits of cross-sectionally derived standards.

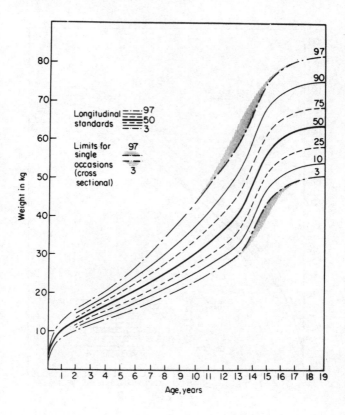

Prepared by Professor J.M. Tanner and Mr R.H. Whitehouse and reproduced by permission of Castlemead Publications, Hertford.

33

GIRLS' HEIGHT

Longitudinal standards for weight attained at given age. The shaded areas represent the 97th and 3rd centile limits of cross-sectionally derived standards.

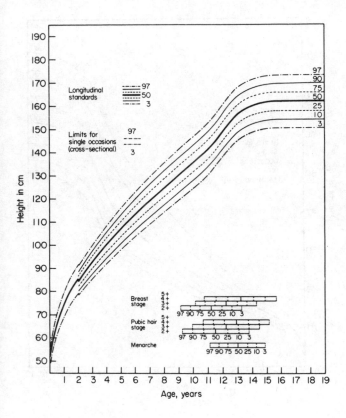

Prepared by Professor J.M. Tanner and Mr R.H. Whitehouse and reproduced by permission of Castlemead Publications, Hertford.

GIRLS' WEIGHT

Longitudinal standards for weight attained at given age. The shaded areas represent the 97th and 3rd centile limits of cross-sectionally derived standards.

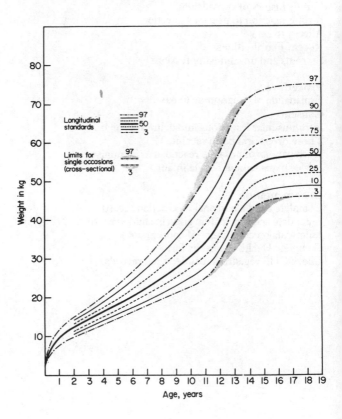

Prepared by Professor J.M. Tanner and Mr R.H. Whitehouse and reproduced by permission of Castlemead Publications, Hertford.

IMMUNISATION OF CHILDREN

History
General health
History of convulsions or cerebral irritability
Family history of convulsions
Strong reaction to previous injection
Allergy to eggs
Recent Febrile Illness
Steroids and immunosuppression

Procedure
Explanation of programme to parents
Consent
Intramuscular injections into deltoid or thigh
Three drops oral polio vaccine
Warn parents of possible reactions to immunisations
Advice management febrile infant

Documentation
Complete child's personal vaccination record
Enter date and vaccination given in child's record card (FP7A)
Enter data on computer—if appropriate
Complete Health Authority form
Check CHS registration and 'target' records

IMMUNISATION OF CHILDREN—continued
Suggested immunisation programme (see pp. 38–45 for notes)

Age	Vaccine	Dose & Route	Notes
2 months	Triple or Dip/Tet Polio (L*)	0.5 ml IM 3 drops, oral	Interval between 1st & 2nd visits not less than 4 weeks
3 months	Triple or Dip/Tet Polio (L*)	0.5 ml IM 3 drops, oral	Interval between 2nd & 3rd visits not less than 4 weeks
4 months	Triple or Dip/Tet Polio (L*)	0.5 ml IM 3 drops, oral	
12–18 months	Measles/Mumps/Rubella (MMR)	0.5 ml IM/SC	
4–5 years	Dip/Tet Polio (L*) MMR	0.5 ml IM 3 drops oral 0.5 ml IM/SC	School entry If not given earlier
10–14 years	Rubella (L*)	0.5 ml SC	Girls only (if not given previously)
10–14 years (or infancy)	BCG	0.1 ml intradermal	Tuberculin negative children only. Interval of 3 weeks between BCG & Rubella
15–18 years	Tetanus Polio (L*)	0.5 ml IM 3 drops oral	School leavers

*Live Vaccine
From *Immunisation against Infectious Disease*, (DHSS) PL CMO (90)3.

IMMUNISATION AGAINST DIPHTHERIA

Indications
Primary immunisation of all children under 10 years
Adults at risk of exposure with positive Schick test

Contraindications
Acute febrile illness
Aged more than 10 (if 25 Lf vaccine is used)
Previous serious reaction

Side effects
Transient
   Fever
   Malaise
   Headaches
   Local reactions

Rarely
   Anaphylactic reactions
   Neurological reactions

Administration
   0.5 ml by deep subcutaneous or intramuscular injection
   25 Lf Diphtheria toxin for children, 1.5 Lf for adults.
   Usually in combination with pertussis and/or tetanus
   3 doses with intervals of 1 month starting at 2 months for children
   3 doses with 1 month intervals for adults

IMMUNISATION AGAINST PERTUSSIS

Indications
All children from 2 months to 6 years, unless contraindicated

Contraindications
Acute febrile illness
History of reaction to a previous dose
History of cerebral irritation or damage as a neonate
History of fits or convulsions
Idiopathic epilepsy in parent or sibling
Development delays
Neurological disease

Side effects
Transient
    Fever
    Malaise
    Screaming
    Drowsiness
    Headache
    Local reactions

Neurological
    Febrile convulsion
    Encephalopathy
    Permanent brain damage

Administration
0.5 ml monovalent vaccine deep subcutaneous or intra-muscular. Usually combined with diphtheria and tetanus
Three doses with intervals of 1 month. Start at 2 months. Not indicated if child is more than 6 years

IMMUNISATION AGAINST TETANUS

Indications

Primary immunisation of children	(2, 3 and 4 months)
Post primary immunisation	(4–5 years)
Reinforcing dose for school leavers	(15–19 years)
Reinforcing dose for all adults	(every 10 years)
Special risk groups; farmers, gardeners	(every 5 years)
Primary immunisation for non-immune adults after sustaining open wounds	(as for children)

Contraindications
Acute febrile illness
Recent tetanus vaccination (less than 1 year)

Side effects
Local injection site reactions (up to 10 days)
Transient
    Headache
    Malaise
    Fever
    Lethargy
    Myalgia
    Urticaria

Anaphylactoid reaction (rare)
Peripheral neuropathy (rare)

Administration
Adsorbed tetanus toxoid (ATT)
0.5 ml vaccine by deep subcutaneous or intramuscular route.
Usually in combination with pertussis and/or diphtheria in children.
3 doses with intervals of 1 month

Human tetanus immunoglobulin (HTIG)

2.5 ml intramuscular	Available in hospital only
Indications	Delay in treating susceptible wound
	Devitalised tissue in wounds
	Puncture wounds
	Evidence of sepsis
	Immunosuppressed patients

IMMUNISATION AGAINST POLIO

Indications

Primary immunisation of all children	(2, 3 and 4 months)
Post-primary immunisation	(4–5 years)
Reinforcing dose for school leavers	(15–19 years)
Special risks as adults	(every 10 years)

Travelling in endemic or epidemic areas

Health care workers in contact with polio cases

Non-immune adults and parents in contact with individuals receiving vaccine

Contraindications (live vaccine)

Acute febrile illness

Steroids, radiation therapy, immunosuppression

Malignancy affecting immunological mechanism

1st trimester of pregnancy

Penicillin allergy (for IPV only)

Administration

Oral polio vaccine (OPV)

3 drops orally as drops on sugar lump.

Usually simultaneously with other primary vaccine in children

Inactivated polio vaccine (IPV)

0.5 ml subcutaneous or intramuscular for those in whom live vaccine is contraindicated

IMMUNISATION AGAINST MEASLES

Indications
All children in their 2nd year (irrespective of a possible history
   of previous measles infection)
Especially children:
   With condition affecting growth
   In residential care
   Starting in playgroup, etc.
Within 3 days of exposure for non-immune contacts
Not routinely indicated for adults

Contraindications (live vaccine)
Acute febrile illness
Steroids, radiotherapy, immunosuppression
Malignancy affecting immunological mechanisms
Pregnancy
Allergy to neomycin or polymyxin
Anaphylactoid reactions to egg protein
History or family history of convulsions
Blood or plasma transfusions or immunoglobulin injection
   within 3 months

Side effects
Reactivation of TB
Subclinical measles infection
Transient fever and malaise (within 10 days)
Anaphylactoid reactions

(The risk of encephalitis and subacute sclerosing encephalitis
is considerably less than with the natural disease.)

Administration
0.5 ml freshly mixed vaccine by deep subcutaneous or
   intramuscular route
Measles immunisation usually given in MMR

IMMUNISATION AGAINST MUMPS

Indications
All children in their 2nd year (as part of MMR)
Susceptible adults

Contraindications
Pregnancy
Acute febrile illness
Steroids, radiotherapy, immunosuppression
Malignancy affecting immunological mechanisms
Allergy to Neomycin or Polymixin
Anaphylactoid reaction to egg protein
Previous severe reaction to mumps or MMR vaccine
Blood or plasma transfusions or immunoglobulin infection
    within 3 months

Side effects
Teratogenesis in pregnant women
Transient
    fever, sore throat, headache
    lymphadenopathy, rashes
    rarely parotid swelling, pruritis, purpura
    arthralgia

Administration
0.5 ml freshly mixed vaccine by deep subcutaneous or
    intra-muscular route
Usually given in MMR

IMMUNISATION AGAINST RUBELLA

Indications
All girls between 10 and 14 years (irrespective of possible history or previous rubella infection) unless known previously immunisation

Non-immune women of child-bearing age (provided they are not pregnant and are using reliable contraception)

All non-immune women working with children (provided that, if of child-bearing age, they are not pregnant and using reliable contraception)

Contraindications (live vaccine)
Pregnancy
Acute febrile illness
Steroids, radiotherapy, immunosuppression
Malignancy affecting immunological mechanisms
Allergy to Neomycin or Polymixin
Allergy to rabbit protein (for 'Condevax')

Side effects
Teratogenesis in pregnant women
Transient
    Fever, sore throat
    Lymphadenopathy rashes
    Arthralgia, peripheral neuropathy (rare)

Administration
0.5 ml of freshly mixed vaccine by deep subcutaneous or intramuscular route
Inform all adult women of their rubella status

IMMUNISATION AGAINST TUBERCULOSIS

Indications
Those with a negative tuberculin test who are:
  Contacts of confirmed cases
  Children from high risk communities
  All neonates from high risk communities
  All health workers
  School children between 10 and 14 years
  Students in higher education

Contraindications (live vaccine)
Acute febrile illness
Dermatitis at injection site
Positive tuberculin test
Pregnancy
Steroids, radiotherapy, immunosuppression
Malignancy affecting immunological mechanisms
Recent administration of other live vaccine (3 weeks)
HIV positive

Side effects
Local reaction including ulcers, abscesses, and lymphadenitis
Anaphylactoid reaction

Administration
Careful intradermal injection of 0.1 ml of BCG vaccine into
  the deltoid region, after carrying out a tuberculin test

IMMUNISATION AGAINST INFLUENZA

Indications
Chronic chest disease
Chronic heart disease
Chronic kidney disease
Diabetes
Immunosuppression

Institutionalised and elderly
Health workers with heavy exposure to influenza

Contraindications
Allergy to eggs, Polymixin and Neomycin
Pregnancy (unless special need)

Side effects
Local skin reaction
Minor flu-like illness
Urticaria (very rare)

Administration
Composition of vaccine is reviewed annually
Vaccine may be 'whole virus', 'split virus' or 'surface antigen'
    and contain 1, 2 or 3 viruses.
Intramuscular or deep subcutaneous injection

COMMON INFECTIOUS DISEASES

Disease	Usual incubation period (days)	Interval between onset of illness and appearance or rash (days)	Minimum period of isolation providing the patient appears well
Chicken pox	10–21	0–2	Seven days from appearance of rash; all the scabs need not have separated
Dysentery (Sonne)	1–7	–	Until 24 hours after cessation of diarrhoea
Infective jaundice	14–42	–	Until clinical recovery
Measles	7–21	3–5	Until clinical recovery
Mumps	12–28	–	Until disappearance of all swelling
Rubella	14–21	0–2	Until clinical recovery
Scarlet fever	2–5	1–2	Until clinical recovery
Whooping cough	5–14	–	Until completion of antibiotics

There is no routine exclusion of contacts of any of these infectious diseases. Exclusion is at the discretion of the doctor, i.e. children are special risk.

Recommended immunisations

Years of immunity given by immunisations.

Immunity given by immunisation	Tetanus	Polio	Cholera	Typhoid	Meningococcal Meningitis	Yellow Fever	Typhus	Hepatitis (& Globulin)
N. Europe & USA	5–10 yr	10 yr						
S. Europe, Middle East	5–10 yr	10 yr	6 m	3 yr				6 week to 6 m
Africa & Far East	5–10 yr	10 yr	6 m	3 yr	3 yr			6 week to 6 m
Central Africa	5–10 yr	10 yr	6 m	3 yr	3 yr	10 yr	1 yr	6 week to 6 m
Central & S. America	5–10 yr	10 yr	6 m	3 yr		10 yr	1 yr	6 week to 6 m
Canada, New Zealand and Australia			6 m					

Cholera vaccine gives limited protection and is often only given if
1) Country requires vaccination for entry
2) Epidemic or special risk
Rabies vaccination not recommended for routine vaccination of travellers unless exposed to specific risk.

IMMUNISATION FOR TRAVELLERS
—continued

Malarial prophylaxis is needed before entering certain countries; start 1 week before travelling; continue for 6 weeks after returning. Consult the BNF or recommendations by the local DHA.

Gamma-globulin injection may be required if travelling to countries where hepatitis is a risk.

Recommendations vary. Advice can be obtained from DHA, Tropical Diseases Hospital, Embassies or International Relations Division, DHSS 01-407-5522, Ex. 6711, or DHSS booklet *Immunisation against Infectious Diseases* (HMSO).

Documentation

Complete any international certificates. State batch no. of vaccines.

Complete FP73 in detail including destination and countries en route.

Enter details including Batch No. and expiry date in patient's notes.

Check certificate is completed fully and signed by patient and yourself.

CONTRAINDICATION TO IMMUNISATION FOR TRAVELLERS

	Anthrax	Cholera	Hepatitis A	Human Normal Immunoglobulin	Hepatitis B	Meningococcal meningitis	Polio	Tetanus	Typhoid	Yellow Fever
Acute infection			•		•	•	•	•	•	
Chronic illness			•						•	
Severe reactions to previous immunisation	•	•	•			•		•		
Steroids, immunosuppression, radiation							•			•
Malignancy or deficiency in immune systems							•			•
Pregnancy						•	•		•	•
Age less than 18 months							•			
Age less than 12 months		•					•		•	
Age less than 9 months		•					•		•	•
Allergy to Neomycin Polymixin										•
Allergy to penicillin							• (IPV)			
Allergy to egg protein										•

IMMUNISATION PROGRAMME

Standard programme

Day	Vaccine	Notes
Day 1	Yellow fever	At yellow fever vaccination centre
	1st Cholera	
	1st Oral polio	
Day 2 or 3	1st Typhoid	
	1st Tetanus	
Day 9 or 10	2nd Cholera	
Day 21 (approx.)	Meningococcal vaccine	
Day 29	2nd Typhoid	If previously immunised against cholera, typhoid, tetanus and polio the relevant 2nd may be omitted
	2nd Tetanus	
	2nd Oral polio	
	Gamma Globulin	Give as close to departure as practicable

Rapid programme

Day 1	Yellow fever, meningococcal vaccine
Day 15	Typhoid and Cholera
	Gamma Globulin

Emergency programme

When departure is within 24–48 hours, and cannot be delayed. There is an increased risk of systemic disturbance and this programme should be avoided if possible.

Day 1	Yellow fever – in the arm
	Typhoid and cholera – in the buttocks
	Gamma Globulin – in opposite buttock
	Meningococcal vaccine

Note. The WHO no longer recommends routine Smallpox vaccination. A Doctor's certificate advising against vaccination may be needed for some countries.

IMPORTED DISEASES

History
Country visited
Time and duration of visit
Itinerary and method of travel
Adequacy of prophylactic immunisation
The nature of anti-malarial and other precautions taken
Any other contacts at risk
Illness among other members of the party

Suggested investigations
Full blood count and ESR
Microscopy of thick and thin blood films
Clotted blood for culture, Widal and V_i agglutinins
Stool specimens for microscopy and culture
Mid-stream urine for microscopy, culture and sensitivity
Chest X-ray

IMPORTED DISEASES —continued

Appearance of imported diseases.

Period	Disease	Countries visited
< 10 days	Endemic Typhus	N. India, Pakistan, SE. Asia, Far East, Pacific, Queensland, Africa
	Dengue Yellow Fever	Tropics, Sub-tropics, Africa, Central and South America
Up to 21 days	Malaria (perhaps longer)	Tropics and Sub-tropics
	Typhoid	Tropics, Sub-tropics, Mediterranean
	Trypanosomiasis	Africa 12°N–25°S
	Schistosomiasis (a) haematobium	Nile, Africa, Iraq, Bombay, Mid and Far East
	(b) mansoni	Nile, Africa, Arabia, Central and South America
	Brucellosis	Worldwide
	Tropical Haemorrhagic Fever	West Africa
> 21 days	Kala-azar	North, East, West Africa, Central America, South America China, East India
	Viral Hepatitis	Worldwide
	Filariasis	Africa, SE. Asia, North Australia, West Indies, South America, Pacific
	Amoebiasis	Tropical and Sub-tropical

NOTIFIABLE DISEASES

The Health Service and Public Health Act 1968 and the Public Health (Infectious Disease) Regulations 1988 require a doctor to notify the local Community Physician (Environmental Health) if a person is suffering from one of the following infectious diseases:

Acute encephalitis
Acute meningitis
Acute poliomyelitis
Anthrax
Cholera
Diphtheria
Dysentery –
    amoebic or bacillary
Food poisoning –
    actual or suspected
Infective Jaundice
Lassa fever
Leprosy
Leptospirosis
Malaria
Marburg Disease
Measles
Meningococcal septicaemia
(without meningitis)

Mumps
Ophthalmia neonatorum
Paratyphoid fever A or B
Plague
Rabies
Relapsing fever
Rubella
Scarlet fever
Smallpox
Tetanus
Tuberculosis
Typhoid fever
Typhus fever
Viral haemorrhagic fever
Viral hepatitis
Whooping cough
Yellow fever

Notification, for which a fee is paid, should be made on a certificate obtainable from the DHA or the local government District Environmental Health Department.

AIDS is not a statutorily notifiable disease but doctors are urged to participate in a voluntary confidential reporting scheme. AIDS cases should be reported on a special AIDS clinical report form in *strict medical confidence* to the Director, PHLS Communicable Disease Surveillance Centre, 61 Colindale Ave, London NW9 5EQ (081 200 6868) or locally from physicians in G.U. Medicine.

Scotland and Northern Ireland
Regulations vary from the above list.

INDUSTRIAL DISEASES

Notifiable diseases

These are a group of diseases which, when they occur in factories, are compulsorily notifiable by doctors and employers to the Health and Safety Executive.

Aniline poisoning
Anthrax
Arsenical poisoning
Beryllium poisoning
Cadmium poisoning
Carbon disulphide
  poisoning
Chrome ulceration
Chronic benzene
  poisoning

Compressed air sickness
Epitheliomatous
  ulceration
Lead poisoning
Manganese poisoning
Mercury poisoning
Phosphorus intoxication
Toxic anaemia
Toxic jaundice

If in doubt consult Employment Medical Advisory Service or local Health and Safety Executive.

'Prescribed' diseases

Compensation is payable under the National Insurance (Industrial Injury) Act 1946. The occupations responsible and the list of prescribed diseases are laid down in the Schedule of the Department of Health and Social Security.

USE OF LABORATORY

It is a DHSS recommendation that all GPs have access to hospital laboratories. Pathologists will provide a domiciliary service on request and will discuss any problems with the doctor.

Supplies
FPC
> Sterile disposable plastic syringes
> Needles

Laboratory
> Lists of normal values
> Lists of appropriate containers
> Request forms
> Suitable packaging
> containers, transport media, swabs

Specimens
Specimens and forms should be similarly labelled with:
> Patient's full name
> Date of birth
> Address
> GP's name and address
> Date and time specimen taken
> NHS or private patient

Full clinical information should be supplied:
> Date of onset
> Symptoms
> Diagnosis
> Relevant treatment
> Hepatitis or high risk warning on card and specimen

Transportation
There are usually arrangements with the local laboratory or alternatively specimens can be delivered by the patient or by first class mail. Post Office regulations demand that specimens be in a sealed receptacle in a strong Post Office approved box with sufficient material to prevent leakage if damaged, and marked 'Fragile – with care' and 'Pathological specimen'.

USE OF LABORATORY – Continued

Public Health Laboratory Service
It serves community physicians, general practitioners, and hospitals with responsibility directly to the Secretary of State for Health and Social Security.

Routine Work – comprehensive bacteriological service
Investigation – epidemiology, prevention and control of infectious disease
Advice – to central and local health authorities
Research

High risk groups
Known infectious disease carriers
Hepatitis A or B, syphilis, or AIDS
Chronic liver disease
Jaundice of unknown origin
Haemodialysis
Haemophilia
Immunosuppressive treatment
Organ transplantation
Drug addiction
Sexual contacts of high risk patients

Procedure
Discuss with laboratory
Doctor should take specimens
Plastic gloves and appropriate protective clothing
Screw-capped containers
Specimen and request form labelled in approved manner
Specimens placed in plastic bag, separate from forms

Disposal of needles and syringes
Make special arrangements with waste disposal authority or hospital for disposal of sharps and contaminated waste

Code of practice
See BMA Code of Practice for sterilisation of instruments and control of cross infection (1989).

Check lists

SCREENING

Criteria for screening (Wilson 1976)
The condition screened for should be an important one
There should be an acceptable treatment for patients with the disease
The facilities for diagnosis and treatment should be available
There should be a recognised latent or early symptomatic stage
There should be a suitable test or examination
The test or examination should be acceptable to the population
The natural history of the condition should be understood
There should be an agreed policy on whom to treat
The cost of case finding should be balanced in relation to civil expenditure on medical care as a whole
Case finding should be a continuing process

Wilson 1976 'Some principles of early diagnosis and detection' Proceedings of the Colloquium, Magdalen College, Oxford 1965 (ed. G. Teeling-Smith), Office of Health Economics, London.

CONTINUING CARE
Case finding
Disease register	Entry criteria
	Screening or case finding
Call and recall system	Computer or manual

Cooperation
Patient compliance	Full discussion
	Shared clinical objectives
	Cooperation cards
	Regular follow up
Primary care colleagues	Administration and secretarial Nurse support Partners role
Consultant colleagues	Shared care and Supportive role Specialist advice Technical backing

Control
Passive/Monitoring	Patient; symptom charts, etc., Doctor; regular recording of objective indicators
Active/Intervention	Patient; Titrate therapy against severity
	Doctor; initiate changes in objectives and management

Complications
Prevention	Advise on preventive measures
	Detect and intervene early with preventable complications
Mitigation	Monitor progress of any unavoidable complications
	Educate to avoid exacerbations
Continuity	Recall regularly
	Review objectives
	Revise protocols
	Renew motivation and rewards
	Reinforce cooperation
	Audit

PSYCHO-SEXUAL HISTORY

Present complaint

Personal history
Childhood and friends
Family inter-relationships
School and achievements
Religious and moral attitudes
Marital history
Extra-marital history

Sexual history
Sex education
Family attitudes and taboos
Traumatic experiences
Puberty
Masturbation
Homosexuality
First sexual experiences
Subsequent sexual experience
Present sexual relationship

Present sexual function
Libido
Arousal
Potency
Ejaculation
Orgasm
Frequency of intercourse
Variations

Past medical history

Past obstetric and gynaecological history

Past psychiatric history

Social history

Drugs

Examination

Investigations

PRE-CONCEPTION CHECK

DISCUSSION

Present family planning
Medical and obstetric history
Family history of both partners
Place of delivery
Role of midwife
Genetic counselling as appropriate, seek specialist advice
Smoking
Alcohol
Drugs e.g. anticonvulsants
  long-term antibiotics
  or immuno-suppressives

Investigation
Blood pressure
Urinalysis
Weight
Rubella titre – and vaccination
Full blood count
Blood group
Rhesus antibodies
Syphilis serology
Hb electrophoresis. Sickle cell and thalassaemia
Breast examination
Pelvic examination and smear

Check lists

SPORTS INJURY

History
Sport
Action causing injury
Severity of injury
Loss of consciousness
Level of performance
Training schedule
Forthcoming fixtures
Protective equipment
Techniques
Previous injuries

Examination
Impairment of function
Bone injury
Soft tissue injury
Visceral injury

Aims of treatment
Appropriate first aid
Restoration of function
Preservation of fitness
Prevention of recurrence
Restoration of confidence

BANNED SUBSTANCES IN SPORT
The International Olympic Committee's Medical Commission
list of Doping Classes and Methods (1989)

I Doping classes
Stimulants to the nervous system
e.g. amphetamines, cocaine, ephedrine
Narcotic analgesics
e.g. codeine, morphine, pethidine
Anabolic steroids
e.g. Stanozolol, testosterone
Beta-blockers
e.g. Propranolol, Atenolol
Diuretics
e.g. frusemide, hydrochlorothiazide, Spironolacetone
Peptide hormones and analogues
e.g. HCCT, ACTH, somatotrophin (LGH)

II Doping methods
Blood doping
Pharmacological, chemical and physical manipulation

BANNED SUBSTANCES IN SPORT—
continued
III Classes of drugs subject to certain restrictions
Alcohol
Marijuana
Local Anaesthetics
Corticosteroids

Treatment guidelines for participants in sport

Cough	Allowed	Steam and menthol inhalation. All antibiotics.
	Banned	Products containing Ephedrine; most proprietary cough syrups.
Hay Fever	Allowed	Antihistamines, steroid nasal sprays. Cromoglycate nasal and eye preparations.
	Banned	Pseudoephedrine, codeine, Dextropropoxyphene.
Asthma	Allowed	Salbutamol, Terbutaline, Cromoglycate, Beclomethasone—by inhaler only.
	Banned	Ephedrine related compounds.
Sore throat	Allowed	Soluble Paracetamol gargle.
Vomiting	Allowed	Electrolyte Rehydrating Solutions.
Diarrhoea	Allowed	Electrolyte Rehydrating Solutions. Loperamide, Diphenoxylate.
	Banned	Products containing codeine or morphine.

Sportsmen and women should be advised to contact their sport's governing body for current comprehensive advice. The rules vary for different sports and lists change. They are responsible for what they take.

The Sports Council produce 'credit cards' listing advice (071 388 1277) (also Sports Councils for Wales and Scotland).

REHABILITATION

Definition
The restoration of patients to their fullest physical, mental and social capability

Areas to consider
Avoidable disability
Physical and mental health
Aids and appliances
Return to work
Community involvement
Self-help groups and support for careers
Sexual activity
Information and health education

Rehabilitation teams may comprise:

Doctors	Occupational Therapist
Health Visitor	Physiotheropist
Nurse	Remedial Gymnast
Social Worker	Speech Therapist
Disablement Resettlement Officer	

Role of GP
Early treatment of disease
Long term medical supervision
Co-ordination of help in the community
Support for patient, family and friends

Rehabilitation of coronary patient
Patient with uncomplicated myocardial infarction will normally be capable of normal range of physical activity, including sexual intercourse, within 4–6 weeks.
Important to avoid long term disability by encouraging activity
Some hospitals now have Coronary Rehabilitation Programmes
Certain occupations are affected by history of myocardial infarction e.g. PSV driver

ASSESSMENT OF THE DISABLED

Medical support
Drug therapy
Nursing care
Occupational therapy
Physiotherapy

Locomotion
Aids to daily living
Sticks, frames and wheelchairs
Tricycle, car and bus

Accommodation
Access
Doors and floors
Bathroom and toilets
Heating and cooking
Warden controlled flat
Part III accommodation

Social support
Name and telephone number of main carer
Food, shopping and laundry
Family and neighbours
Home help
Meals on wheels
Societies
Clubs and churches
Day care centres
Voluntary organisations
Financial help

ASSESSMENT OF THE ELDERLY

The new GP contract places an obligation on doctors to offer a
consultation and domiciliary visit to patients aged 75 years and
over. The assessment covers
(a) Sensory function
(b) Mobility
(c) Mental condition
(d) Physical condition including continence
(e) Social Environment
(f) use of medicines
The following check list is more comprehensive:

Risk factors
Extreme age
Chronic illness
Immobility
Loneliness
Recent bereavement
Poverty

Medical assessment
Weight, BP, urine
Teeth and dentures
Sight and hearing
Bowel and bladder function
Drug regimen
Assessment for dependency

Psychiatric assessment
Intellectual function
Orientation and memory
Psychiatric symptoms
Social crises

ASSESSMENT OF THE ELDERLY—continued

Accommodation
Access
Stairs and alterations
Heating and lighting
Bathroom and toilets
Housework and hygiene
Laundry and shopping
Cooking and diet
Part III accommodation

Social support
Family and neighbours
Health visitors and social workers
Bath attendant and chiropodist
Helping agencies, disease societies and self-help groups
Day care
Hospital arrangements
Finance, pensions and benefits

FITNESS TO DRIVE

Patients over 70 require 3-yearly medical certificates.

The patient, holding or applying for a licence, is himself obliged to notify the Licensing Authority if he is suffering from a relevant or prospective disability.

The doctor should act as adviser to his patient. He should use his own discretion in informing the Licensing Authority if he thinks that the driving of a patient could be a danger. A medical defence society should be consulted if there is a potential breach of confidence.

History
Driving habits: local, rush hour, professional, experience
Coronary, heart disease, aortic valve disease
Diabetic hypoglycaemia
Epilepsy
Transient cerebral ischaemia, Ménières disease
Vertigo, Parkinsonism, multiple sclerosis
Limb disability
Severe deafness
Monocular vision, diplopia, night blindness
Subnormality, illiteracy, psychiatric breakdown
Dementia
Drugs

Examination
Heart rate, heart sounds, blood pressure
Power, co-ordination, sensation
Visual acuity, fields and fundi
Hearing

Investigation
Urine, ECG, if indicated

The doctor must refer to the current guidelines* on medical requirements for different licences.

*See Consulting Room Bookshelf, p. 224

TRAVEL BY AIR –
CONTRAINDICATIONS

Cardiovascular disease
Myocardial infarction (within 6 weeks of onset)
Uncompensated cardiac failure. Patients with angina or
  controlled cardiac failure may be carried but extra oxygen
  will be supplied
Recent cerebral infarction
Severe anaemia including sickling disorders

Respiratory tract
Severe otitis media or sinusitis, or recent middle ear surgery
  or eustachian catarrh
Pneumothorax
Irreversible airways disease
Within 21 days of major chest surgery

Gastrointestinal
Within 10 days of simple abdominal operation
Within 3 weeks of G.I. haemorrhage
Colostomies are acceptable if extra dressings are carried

Central nervous system
Epilepsy – acceptable if extra anti-convulsants are carried
Mental illness if without escort and sedation

Diabetes
Diabetic passengers may travel if they manage their own
  medication. Special diets provided. Note time zone change
  on arrival at destination

Infectious diseases

Pregnancy
Beyond 35 weeks gestation for international journeys and 36
  weeks gestation for short flights

Air in body cavities
Introduction of air to body cavities for diagnostic or
  therapeutic purposes within 7 days

Fractured mandible with wiring

HEALTH CHECKS

The new GP contract introduces New Registration Health
Checks and Health Checks for patients not seen by any doctor
within the preceding 3 years.

    Current state of health
    Past medical history
    Family history
    Medication (including oral contraceptive use*)
    Allergies
    Immunisations
    Tests for breast and cervical cancer
    Social history (employment, housing, family circumstances)
    Lifestyle (diet, exercise, smoking, alcohol, misuses of drugs
       and solvents)
Examination
    Height
    Weight
    Ideal weight*
    Blood pressure
    Urine test (protein and glucose)
    Record results
    Assessment of medical needs
    Advice as appropriate
    Referral as appropriate
Opportunistic Preventive Care
    Cervical cytology*
    Breast examination*
    Immunisation*
    Cholesterol estimation*
    Consider recall frequency if at increased risk*

*Not required in Terms of Service

ABBREVIATIONS

ACBS	Advisory Committee on Borderline Substances
AHCPA	Association of Health Centre and Practice Administrators
AMS	Association of Medical Secretaries
AMSPAR	Association of Medical Secretaries, Practice Administrators and Receptionists
BMA	British Medical Association
BNF	British National Formulary
CAB	Citizens' Advice Bureau
CHC	Community Health Council
CSM	Committee for the Safety of Medicines
DHA	District Health Authority
DHSS	Department of Health and Social Security
FHSA	Family Health Services Authority (was Family Practitioner Committee, FPC)
GPFC	General Practice Finance Corporation
GMSC	General Medical Services Committee
HEA	Health Education Authority
HVA	Health Visitors' Association
JCPTGP	Joint Committee on Postgraduate Training for General Practice
LMC	Local Medical Committee
MDU	Medical Defence Union
MIMS	Monthly Index of Medical Specialties
MPC	Medical Practices Committee
MPS	Medical Protection Society
MRC	Medical Research Council
MWF	Medical Womens Federation
NCC	National Consumer Council
NIC	National Insurance Contribution
PPA	Prescription Pricing Authority
PPG	Patient Participation Group
RCGP	Royal College of General Practitioners
RCN	Royal College of Nursing
RHA	Regional Health Authority
RMO	Regional Medical Officer
SFA	Statement of Fees and Allowances ('The Red Book')
SMP	Statutory Maternity Pay
SSP	Statutory Sick Pay

STRUCTURE OF THE NHS

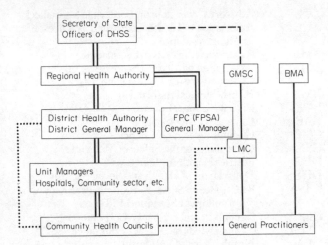

Key

(════════) Accountable/in contract with

(. . . . .) Co-opted representation

(─────) Elected representation

(– – – – –) Negotiates

Current developments will alter this structure, for example the replacement of FPC/FPSA with the new Family Health Services Authority.

STRUCTURE OF THE FPC

FPCs are becoming FHSAs. Details of structure and nomenclature will vary.

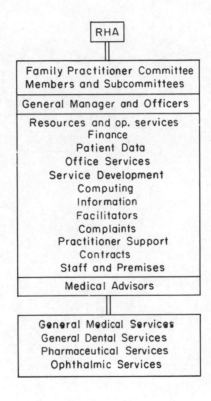

EDUCATIONAL COMMITTEES
(VOCATIONAL TRAINING)

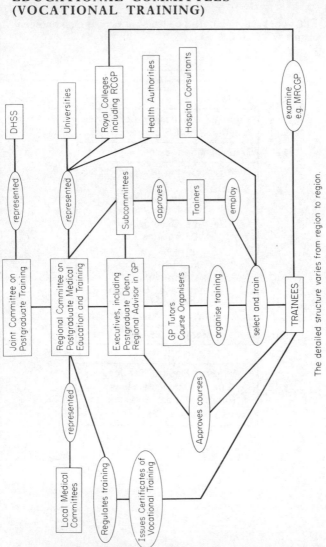

The detailed structure varies from region to region.

MEDICO - POLITICAL COMMITTEES

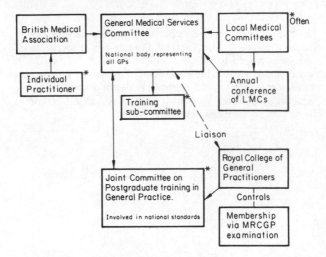

*Representation by GP trainees. There may be local variations.

THE REGIONAL MEDICAL SERVICE OF THE DHSS

The Regional Medical Service has been radically changed with the new contract. The General Practitioner responsibilities have been passed to FHSA Medical Advisors. Some RMOs have continued within the field of Social Security, providing independent refereeing when there is doubt about a patient's capability for work. Decisions are based on reports from doctors and clinical examinations.

ORGANISATION OF SOCIAL SERVICES

Social services Departments are run by local authorities and vary from area to area. A department will be divided by functions

Research, Development and Training

Personnel

Administration and Finance

Domiciliary Social Work. General Medical and Psychiatric Social Workers. Area Offices

Domiciliary Support Services. Home helps, Meals on Wheels, voluntary services

Care Services—residential and day care

Northern Ireland
Health & Social Services are integrated.

PATIENT PARTICIPATION GROUPS (PPG)

Patient participation groups are local and autonomous groups of patients. Their aim is to improve primary care by supporting their primary care team, to promote mutual trust, and to co-ordinate consumer activities:

Feedback on existing services
Accessibility
Acceptability
Responsiveness to need
Effectiveness

Feedback for planning new services

Complaints/grievances/suggestions

Health education
Specialist lectures
Education on health beliefs
Leaflets, posters, audiovisual aids
Use of media

Support of primary health care
Transport
Prescription collection

Self-help groups

Community care
Elderly
Young mothers
Disabled
Social events
Communications

Lobbying outside bodies
Health Authorities
Local Government
Central Government

78

HELPING AGENCIES

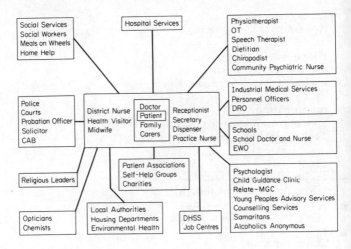

REASONS FOR REFERRAL

Emergency care
Assessment and management

Diagnosis
Expert second opinions
Exclusion of suspected pathology

Investigation
Specialist knowledge (e.g. Immunopathology)
Technical facilities (e.g. X-rays)

Treatment
Technical skills and facilities
    (e.g. surgery, chemotherapy)
Specialist skills
    (e.g. psychiatry, dermatology)

Continuing care
Advice on symptom control
Assessment of complications

Doctor: patient relationship
New initiatives in 'difficult cases'
Patient's request for a second opinion

STANDARD REFERRAL LETTER

To be effective a letter to a consultant should be brief. It should include the detailed information that he may not be able to obtain from the patient himself.

Name, age, address
Marital status, occupation, hospital number

Reason for referral
Opinion or action requested
Degree of urgency

Time scale of events
Relevant personal and family history
Relevant findings on examination and investigation

Drug regimen
Drug idiosyncrasies
Patient compliance
Social factors
What the patient has been told
Future management

REFERRAL LETTERS — SPECIAL CASES

In certain circumstances special information will be of value to the hospital staff in addition to the standard referral letter.

Obstetric—see page 18.

Paediatric
Pregnancy and parental attitude to pregnancy
Neonatal and developmental history
History of family dynamics
History or suspicion of child abuse

Sterilisation or vasectomy
Origin of request
Doctor's opinion
Obstetric and gynaecological history
Contraceptive history
Stability of relationship

Termination of pregnancy
History of present pregnancy – LMP gestation
Obstetric and gynaecological history
Medical and psychiatric history
Reasons for request
Patient and family's attitude
Doctor's recommendation
Documentation

Overdose—see page 209

Psychiatric
Full details of present illness and associated disorders
Change in personality or intellect
Previous psychiatric illnesses
Past medical history
Drugs and alcohol
Personal and social history
Family psychiatric illness
Family background

EMERGENCY PSYCHIATRIC ADMISSIONS

Under the 1983 Mental Health Act, an application can be made for compulsory admission 'where the patient is suffering from a mental disorder warranting detention for their own health or safety or for the protection of others'.

Section 2
Compulsory admission for 28 days for 'assessment'
Application by next of kin or approved social worker
Recommendation by two doctors
Contact duty psychiatrist and social worker and arrange home visit

Section 3
Compulsory admission for 6 months for 'treatment'
Application by approved social worker or nearest relative
Recommendation by two doctors
Contact duty psychiatrist and social worker

Section 4
'Emergency' admission for 72 hours for assessment
Application by approved social worker or nearest relative
Recommendation by one doctor

Notes. The social worker is responsible for all documentation and the transport of the patient to hospital.

Scotland and Ireland
The Mental Health Act (Scotland) 1960 provides for compulsory admission under Section 24. The application is made by the nearest relative or mental welfare officer together with a medical recommendation, which must be approved by the Sheriff. In an emergency Section 31 allows the patient to be detained for 7 days.

NON-ACCIDENTAL INJURIES TO CHILDREN—I PHYSICAL ABUSE

History
Declared anxiety of battering
Inappropriate, devious or changing story
Varying reports from different witnesses
Delay in seeking help
Previous unexplained injury
Identify risk factors
    Changes in doctors
    Repeated visits by an anxious mother with a child
    Separation from parents including neonatal period
    Parents subjected to battering
    Social circumstances
    Mental illness in parents
    No helping relatives or friends
    Unrealistic expectations of child
    Apathy or lack of concern for child

Examination
Bruises including petechiae, repetitive bruising, finger and thumb prints, bruises from adult bites
Fractures without a history of accident (radiological appearances include multiple fractures and various stages of healing)
Burns and scalds including cigarette burns
Mouth bruising and lacerations
Skull – fractures, subdural haematoma, retinal haemorrhages
Visceral injuries
General neglect

Action
Health visitor
Social worker
Community physician
Paediatric unit
Place of safety
Police as appropriate

NON-ACCIDENTAL INJURIES
TO CHILDREN—2 SEXUAL ABUSE

Allegations of abuse. Particularly serious if spontaneous.
Sexually provocative to adults.
Unusually detailed knowledge of sexual matters.
Preoccupation with sexual fantasies and behaviour.
Response to questioning by describing sexual abuse.
Specific fears especially of male adult.
Unexplained behavioural or emotional disturbance.
Suspicious family setting.

Lower genito urinary tract symptoms.
G-U injuries or abnormalities.
Faecial soiling retention, rectal bleeding
Rectal abnormalities
Sexually transmitted disease
Pregnancy under 16 years especially where no knowledge of
    identity of father

Full examination and full interview should usually be carried
out by those specially trained.

Action as NAIC

PROBLEM FAMILIES

Persistent truancy
Juvenile delinquency
Probation Order
Care Order
Child Guidance Clinic
Prolonged separation from parents
Repeated hospital treatment
Repeated accidents

Size of family
Maternal age
Family history
Single parent – divorced or separation
Marital problems
Prolonged mental or physical illness
Employment
Finance and benefits
Alcohol, gambling, sex and violence
Criminal record
Suspected child abuse

Housing
Personal and domestic hygiene
Domestic mismanagement
Helping agencies

BODILY ASSAULT

This examination is best conducted by a police surgeon and will involve a written report and possible court appearance.

Procedure
Consent
Chaperone
Suitable premises and lighting
Detailed account of all findings
Photograph or drawing where appropriate
Claim appropriate fee and mileage

History
Date, time, place of incident
Course of events, persons involved, witnesses
Loss of consciousness
Previous medical history
Drugs
Alcohol

Examination
General appearance
Inspect clothing
General examination
Careful examination of any injuries
Age of bruising
Neurological examination

Investigations
X-rays where appropriate
The police will specify what samples are required for the
    forensic laboratory

Check lists

SEXUAL ASSAULT

This examination is best conducted by a police surgeon and will involve a written report and possible court appearance.

Procedure
Written consent from victim, parents or guardian
Chaperone
Suitable premises and lighting
Change of clothing for victim
Establish that sexual intercourse has occurred
Detailed account of all findings
Claim appropriate fee and mileage

History
Date, time, place of incident
Course of events, persons involved, witnesses
Resistance by victim
Menstrual history

Examination
General appearance and behaviour
Apparent age
Inspect clothing
General examination
Nails
Genitalia
Pubic hair

Investigations
Venous blood
Swabs for semen
Clothing fragments
Foreign hairs
Dried blood
The police will specify what samples are required for the forensic laboratory

INTOXICATION WITH ALCOHOL

A doctor is usually only required to take a venous blood sample. The kit is provided by the police. Verbal consent should be obtained.

When examination is required, first obtain written consent.

History
Medical history
Psychiatric history
Previous personality
Medication
Drug abuse

Examination
General appearance and behaviour
Careful examination of any injuries
Mouth and breath
Pulse, blood pressure
Temperature
Skin
Ears and hearing
Eyes
Gait, co-ordination, stance
Mental state, memory
Writing ability

Investigations
Breath test
Urine
Blood for alcohol and drug levels
Blood sugar
Prepare written report and keep copy
Claim fee and mileage from police

Check lists

CORONER'S CASE

Death due to suspected unnatural cause
Cause of death uncertain
No medical attendance in previous fourteen days
Previous accident or injury
Allegations of negligence
Industrial disability or war pension
Alcoholism or self neglect
Death of infant or fostered child
Death due to drugs, poisons or medical treatment
Death due to abortion unless spontaneous
Death in custody or prison
Death in road traffic accident
Death due to factory accident
Suicide

The coroner will issue death certificate, request post-mortem and sign cremation forms.

Scotland
In Scotland the Procurator-Fiscal acts instead of the Coroner.

There is no compulsion to notify death in Scotland except in the case of fatal accidents and death in suspicious circumstances.

The public inquest in England has its counterpart in the Scottish precognition, which is conducted in private by the Procurator-Fiscal.

An exception to this rule is that fatal accidents in Scotland are statutorily made the subject of a public enquiry, conducted by the Sheriff with a jury of seven.

COT DEATH. (SUDDEN INFANT DEATH SYNDROME)

Frequency: One in 500
More common in boys than girls
More common in winter
Usually first 6 months of life, most within 1 year
Less common in breast fed babies

Action to take
As in sudden death. i.e. Establish death has occurred
Identify deceased
Examine body thoroughly, to exclude non-accidental death
    e.g. bruises, petechiae, burns, fractures
History from parents, symptoms, feeding habits, drugs given
Inform coroner
Coroner's officer deals with removal of body
Remove any drugs belonging to child

Leave address of:
Foundation for Study of Infant Deaths,
    5th Floor,
    Grosvenor Place,
    London SW1A 7HD
    Tel. 071-245-9421
    Evenings 081-748-7768

Follow up family
Listen and talk to parents and siblings
Involve Health Visitor in support of family
Advise mother on suppression of lactation if necessary
Discussion of grief and future pregnancies
Consider night sedation for parents if wanted or appropriate

Support groups
Local Paediatric Departments and Social Services Departments will usually know of support schemes locally.

SUDDEN DEATH

Procedure
Identify deceased
Establish that death has occurred
Ascertain cause of death
Discover circumstances from witnesses
Consider consulting colleagues or records
Consider informing police or coroner
Consider the removal of the body
Inform and discuss with relatives
Issue Death Certificate if possible

Police report
Limit report to information requested
Only record observed facts
Use drawings or photographs as appropriate
Make personal notes immediately
Do not interfere with police work

  Brief statement of circumstances
  Confirmation of death
  Identity of deceased
  Rigor mortis and body temperature
  Possible cause of death
  Position of body and state of clothing
  Record of other relevant features
  Retain any blood, tablets, vomitus

KIDNEY DONOR

Ideal	Acceptable
Aged 5 to 50 years	Aged 3 to 60 years

Brain death from:
  Cerebral trauma
  Cerebral haemorrhage
  Proven primary brain tumour
  Cardiac arrest, cause known
	All deaths without transmissible disease

Supported by a ventilator until the kidneys are removed as planned procedure	Most patients maintained on ventilators Death in circumstances which allow the kidneys to be removed and preserved within 45 minutes of cardiac arrest
Normal renal function and blood pressure No past history of either renal disease or hypertension	Moderate renal failure (blood urea less than 12 mmol/1) from either prerenal factors or tubular necrocis Oliguria for less than four hours Hypotension (systolic BP less than 80 mm Hg in an adult) for less than four hours Any kidney without transmissible disease which is capable of supporting life for five years
Exclude: AIDS or Hepatitis B antigenaemia before kidney is used	**Exclude:** AIDS or Hepatitis B antigenaemia before kidney is used
Sepsis	Generalized but not localized sepsis, e.g. bronchial aspirate
Malignancy other than primary brain tumour	Malignancy other than primary brain tumour

BLOOD DONOR

Contraindications

Systemic illness including AIDS, anaemia, asthma, blood dyscrasias, brucellosis, cancers, diabetes, epilepsy, glandular fever, hay fever, heart disease, hypertension, jaundice, kidney disease, malaria, syphilis, stroke, tuberculosis, AIDS risk (including sexual contact HIV positive)

Any medication (wait 3 days following aspirin ingestion; donors on OC pills and HRT usually accepted)

Females under 8 stone in weight

Drug addiction

Disabled people in wheelchairs (owing to insurance cover)

Pregnancy (delay until baby is a year old)

Any infectious disease (within 2 years)

Any infectious disease contact (within 6 months)

Any vaccination (within 6 months)

Any major surgery (within 6 months (minimum))

Any minor surgery (within 1 month)

Earpiercing, tattooing or acupuncture (within 6 months)

Treatment with Human Growth Hormone (at any time)

Receiving blood transfusion (within 6 months)

Recent travel/residence abroad (within 6 months)

Detailed advice—contact local NBTS

Medicine and the law

CONSENT

Any treatment delivered without the consent of a patient is an assault, which may lead to an action for damages.

Consent may be either expressed (in writing or by word of mouth) or implied. The patient or a legally competent deputy should give *written* consent in the following circumstances:

Diagnostic procedures
Therapeutic procedures
Insurance examinations
Provision of medical reports
Research
Post mortem examinations
Bequest of tissues
Cases involving litigation or police

It is imperative that appropriate explanation is given to the patient regarding the proposed procedure and the onus rests with the practitioner to determine the capability of the patient to give valid consent.

In an emergency, where urgent treatment is required or the patient is unconscious, consent should be obtained from a near relative. Failing this the practitioner should render any treatment that he considers immediately necessary.

CONFIDENTIALITY

Confidentiality is implicit in the doctor-patient relationship. Breach of confidence is treated as professional misconduct by the General Medical Council.

Young patient

Patients below the age of 16 should normally have parental consent to all procedures. Certain circumstances may make this inadvisable or unsafe. Consider advice from colleagues or a defence society as appropriate.

Contraception under 16 years—see p. 17.

Confidence of family and friends

It is the right of the patient, whether dead or alive, to keep his confidences with doctors secret from his family or friends if he so wishes.

Statutory duties

A doctor must report infectious and industrial diseases, and also births, stillbirths and deaths. He must return NHS records to the FPC on request but this does not include correspondence.

A doctor has a duty to give information to the police, on request, in relation to certain serious offences under the Road Traffic Act; the doctor should give only the patient's name and address, but no clinical details.

The prevention of Terrorism Act makes it an offence to fail to disclose information about terrorists.

Order of court

Refusal of a doctor to disclose confidential information on request may be in contempt of court. A doctor should first express reluctance to permit a breach of confidence. He should then request permission not to do so, or to do so only in writing.

Protection of the community

A patient, such as an epileptic driver, should first be encouraged to take appropriate action himself. If the doctor takes the initiative a defence society should first be consulted.

RECORDS AND RESPONSIBILITIES

Contractual duty

A GP has a contractual duty to keep proper records, for both legal and medical reasons. In the NHS, these should be on the forms provided by the Family Health Services Authority. The records are owned by the Secretary of State.

Disclosure of records

Disclosure of records can be ordered by the courts not only when the doctor is directly involved, but a litigant can call for the production of his medical records if he is taking action against someone else and requires medical evidence to support his claim.

Disclosure of computerised information is governed by the Data Protection Act.

Vicarious liability

The evolution of the extended 'primary health care team' and computers has created new problems of professional confidence. The practitioner must decide to which team members and in what circumstances the medical records should be available. It must be stressed to all staff that any information they acquire about patients must be treated in absolute confidence.

ACCESS TO MEDICAL REPORTS ACT 1988

This applies to reports by medical practitioners for employment or insurance purposes and does not apply in Northern Ireland, the Channel Islands or the Isle of Man.

Insurance companies or employers may not apply for a medical report unless the patient has given written consent.

The doctor should be sent a copy of the consent which should state whether the patient wishes to see the report.

If the patient does not wish to see the report, the form should be completed and sent to the insurance company or employer. A copy must be kept. The patient has a right during the next 6 months to see the report and obtain a copy of it for which the doctor may charge a reasonable fee.

If the patient wishes to see the report the insurance company or employer should have informed the patient that the doctor has been contacted. The patient has 21 days to make an appointment to see the report or request a copy for which the doctor can make a reasonable charge. Before giving consent for the report to be sent to the insurance company or employer, the patient may ask for the report to be amended, or, if the doctor is unwilling, for a statement of his/her views to be attached to the report.

If the patient has requested to see the report but has not contacted the doctor within 21 days, the report may be sent to the insurance company or employer.

Copies should be kept of all reports.

Under certain circumstances, the doctor may withhold part or all of the report, but the patient should be informed. If in doubt the doctor should consult his/her Medical Defense Organisation.

PRESCRIBING

Registration with the GMC enables a practitioner to prescribe, possess and dispense drugs. The British National Formulary is published jointly by the BMA and the Pharmaceutical Society and gives full guidance on all aspects of prescribing. However, the following information may be of value.

The prescription

The prescriber has a legal responsibility for the drug prescribed even when acting on another's recommendation.

All prescriptions must be signed by hand.

All alterations must be initialled.

The 'NP' box (*Nomen Propium*) on the FP10 if deleted will indicate to the dispenser that no name is to be written on the label.

Any prescription should include:

Patient's name and address – and age if under 12 years

Name of the drug

Dosage – use values above 1, e.g. 500 mg and not 0.5 g

Frequency of dosage

Total dose and volume – form and strength of preparation to be dispensed

Signature and date

Name and address of prescriber.

The date the drugs are dispensed

The words 'keep out of reach of children' (or similar)

The address and telephone number of the dispensing partnership or pharmacy.

PRESCRIBING—continued

Labelling of containers

When dispensing drugs the label of the container should state:

The name of the preparation – if NP box is not deleted, or if NP box is not initialled in the case of a controlled drug. Alternatively, as a description according to the wording of the prescription.

The strength or concentration of the preparation.

The name of the patient.

The name of the Dispensing Partnership or Pharmacy.

Patient information

Name, dosage and timing of medicine

Storage and disposal of medicine

Expected cure or symptom relief

Degree of compliance necessary

Planned duration of treatment

Warning of potential side effects

Warning of potential interactions

Product liability

All doctors ('dispensing' or not) must ensure that the manufacturer or importer of any drug they supply is identifiable, otherwise they may be considered to be the producer and be liable for any damage resulting from the product, irrespective of any negligence.

These rules apply to 'free samples' and drugs given from the black bag.

Adhere strictly to the labelling rules

Record supply in patient's notes

Proprietary drugs—brand name

Generic drugs—manufacturer and supplier

Batch number

Expiry date

Keep records (invoices etc.) and source of supply of all products (for 11 years).

PRESCRIBING CONTROLLED DRUGS

It is an offence to issue an incomplete prescription for a controlled drug and a pharmacist may not dispense such a prescription. The legal requirements under the Misuse of Drugs Regulations 1973 are that such prescriptions be:

Indelibly handwritten, signed and dated by the prescriber and include:
    Other information as p. 99
    Total quantity of drug in words and figures.
These requirements also apply to barbiturates

NHS PRESCRIBING
Certain drugs are not allowed to be prescribed on forms FP10 although they can still be prescribed privately.
A 'black list' is published by the DHSS and this lists all the products which are not available.
MIMS clearly marks drugs which are not available under the NHS or only available generically under the NHS.

DRUGS FOR USE ABROAD
Drugs to be used abroad should be prescribed privately. Controlled drugs cannot be prescribed for patients leaving the country. It is an offence to carry controlled drugs abroad without a licence issued by the Secretary of State.

ACBS PRESCRIPTIONS
Some foods and toilet preparations may be prescribed under the NHS for conditions approved by The Advisory Committee on Borderline Substances. Such prescriptions should be endorsed ACBS.

MISUSE OF DRUGS REGULATIONS

The four schedules relate to the regulations governing the use of drugs.

The three classes relate to the harmfulness of the drugs and the degree of penalty if the drugs are misused.

Schedule 1
Exempts some common preparations containing codeine, dihydrocodeine, pholcodine, medicinal opium or morphine, cocaine and diphenoxylate from the stringent controls of Schedule 2.

Schedule 2
Imposes special requirements for prescribing cocaine, heroin, morphine (see above). Full dispensing record must be kept. Drugs must be kept in locked receptacle.

Schedule 3
Includes amphetamine derivatives. The requirements for Schedule 2 apply, but a register is not required.

Schedule 4
Special licence is required to prescribe this group of drugs which includes LSD, cannabis and other hallucinogens.

Class A
Includes morphine, opium, heroin, methadone, pethidine, cocaine, LSD, and injectable amphetamines.

Class B
Includes oral amphetamines, cannabis, codeine, pholcodine and phenmetrazine.

Class C
Includes methaqualaine and amphetamine derivatives.

PRESCRIBING FOR ADDICTS

A practitioner must have a special licence from the Home Secretary to prescribe the following drugs to addicts.

cocaine	dextromoramide
diamorphine	opium
morphine	methadone
dipipanone	oxycodone

Any of these drugs may be prescribed to addicts if there is an underlying organic disease.

NOTIFICATION OF ADDICTS

The Home Office keeps a register of those addicted to heroin, morphine, cocaine, pethidine, methadone, dextromoramide, dipipanone, and levorphanol.

The GP has access to this register by writing to the Chief Medical Officer or phoning 071-212-0335 or 071-212-6071.

A GP must notify the Chief Medical Officer of any person suspected to be addicted to the above drugs within 7 days. (Address: Drugs Branch, Romney House, Marsham Street, London SW1).

Notification must include:

Name and address of patient
Sex and date of birth
NHS number
Date of first attendance
Name(s) of the drug(s) of addiction.

Scotland and Northern Ireland
Notification to the Chief Medical Officer, Ministry of Health and Social Services, Dundonald House, Belfast.

In Scotland, drug addicts have to be notified to the Scottish Home and Health Department.

103

THERAPEUTIC ABORTION

The Abortion Act 1967 allows for two medical practitioners to certify the need for termination of pregnancy under the following circumstances:

1   That continuation of the pregnancy would involve risk to the life of the pregnant woman greater than if the pregnancy were terminated.
2   That it would involve risk of injury to the physical or mental health of the pregnant woman greater than if the pregnancy were terminated.
3   That it would involve risk of injury to the physical or mental health of any existing children of the pregnant woman's family greater than if the pregnancy were terminated.
4   That there is a substantial risk that if the child were born it would suffer from physical or mental abnormalities so as to be seriously handicapped.

There are exceptions to the above rules:
The operation and termination may be performed by a practitioner who forms the opinion in good faith that the termination is necessary, as an emergency, to save life or prevent grave permanent injury to the patient.

THERAPEUTIC ABORTION–Continued

Forms
Form HSA1 (green) signed by two medical practitioners to be kept in the patient's notes.

Form HSA2 signed by one medical practitioner for the emergency situation.

Form HSA3 (buff) is a notification of the operation and is sent to the DHSS and kept by them.

Place of termination
This must be an NHS hospital or an approved place.

Consent
This must be obtained from the patient. The husband's consent is not required legally.

With girls between sixteen and twenty-one years of age no consent is needed from the parents legally, but with the girl's permission, it is prudent to obtain their consent.

If the girl is under sixteen years of age and her wishes differ from those of her parents, then a defence society should be consulted.

Scotland and Northern Ireland
In Northern Ireland the Act does not apply.
In Scotland the forms are different for therapeutic abortion.

BEQUEST AND TRANSPLANTATION

Anatomy Act 1832
Those wishing to bequeath their bodies for dissection should be advised to contact the Professor of Anatomy at the nearest Medical School (in London, HM Inspector of Anatomy).

Human Tissues Act 1961
There are two ways organs can be obtained for transplant purposes:
1 'Contracting out'. After reasonable enquiry to exclude any objection by the deceased's relatives (or the deceased before death), the person in lawful possession of the body may authorise the use of any part of it for medical purposes.
2 'Contracting in'. When the deceased expressed the wish, the person in lawful possession of the body may accede to his request.

The consent of HM Coroner is required if an inquest is ordered, or is likely.

Corneal Grafting Act 1952
This Act permits the removal of eyes shortly after death in cases where the deceased had expressed willingness during life and the relatives are in agreement. Contact RNIB, 224 Great Portland Street, London W1.

WILLS

A doctor may be asked to examine a person who wishes to make a will to ascertain whether his mental state will permit a reasoned disposal of his property. He should only witness a patient's will if he is prepared to testify later to that patient's testamentary capacity. The patient should know what property he possesses and which people should reasonably benefit. He should know that he is making a will. As a witness the doctor will forego any legacy which might be received from the will.

SOLICITOR'S REPORT

Establish the purpose of the report and who is requesting it.
Write clearly and in layman's terms.
Information should relate only to questions asked.
   Hearsay evidence in a chronological account
   Patient's treatment and progress
   Objective findings
   Opinions on suffering and prognosis should be as objective
      as possible.
Retain a copy of the report for six years.
Statement of a proper fee.

WITNESS IN COURT

Seek advice of Medical Defence Organisation

Establish what is expected in court
Establish what category of witness is required
    Expert   – with specialist knowledge
    Professional – with particular knowledge of the case under
                   discussion
    Ordinary   – with a citizen's responsibilities
Opinions previously given in written statements may be read
    out in court
Refer to notes made at the time with permission of the court
Remain as impartial as possible
Answer only what is asked and in simple language
Confine answers to fact rather than opinion
Admit to ignorance rather than elaborating the answers
Claim the appropriate statutory fee or negotiate the fee
    beforehand

The primary health care team

Aims
Health maintenance
Illness prevention
Assessment and management of illness
Rehabilitation
Supportive care

The 'nuclear team'
General practitioner
Treatment room sister
Dispenser
Receptionist
Practice manager
Health visitor
Community midwife
District nursing sister

The 'extended team'
Social worker
Care assistant
Home help
Family aid
Counsellor
Community psychiatric nurse
Geriatric health visitor
Chiropodist
Dietitian
Occupational therapist
Physiotherapist
Speech therapist
School nurse
School medical officer

TREATMENT ROOM SISTER or 'PRACTICE NURSE'

Employed by the practice or DHA. May require further training or supervision. The role may be extended to include:

Primary assessment	First contact, telephone advice
First aid and SRN	Accidents, dressings
procedures	Bandages, splints, plasters
	Infra-red treatment, syringing ears
	Assisting doctors, hospital liaison
	Allergy tests, audiograms
	Venepuncture, urinalysis, ECG
Minor operations	Suturing, warts, pessary changes
	Injections and abscesses
Clinics	Health checks and assessment
	Diabetic, Hypertension
	Asthma, Cytology
	Obesity, Family planning
	Well-woman
Immunisations	Information, advice
	Assessment and injection
Health education	Information (patients and lay staff)
	Notice-board display
	Dietary and exercise advice
Counselling	
Stock-taking	Supplies dressings and drugs
and ordering	
Maintenance and	Surgical equipment
renewal	Resuscitation equipment,
	Laundry
	Disposal of sharps and clinical waste
Dispensing	

PRACTICE MANAGER

Employed by the practice or District Health Authority

Duties
Patients
Recognise patient's needs and wants
Patient Participation Group liaison
Complaints
Quality control

Primary health care team
Communication
Meetings and minutes
Welfare
Team development
Duty rotas

Liaison
Regional Health Authority, District Health Authority,
Family Practitioner Committee
Accountants and solicitors
Visitors

Training
New Practice Managers
Reception staff in-service training
New staff induction
Health education
Personal development

Administration
Health and Safety Officer
Book-keeping and accounts
Pensions, PAYE, SSP, SMP, NIC
Audit and statistics
Computer supervision
Quarterly and annual reports
Stock-taking and equipment
Premises—furnishings and up-keep

RECEPTION STAFF

Employed by the practice or District Health Authority

Duties

Reception desk
First contact with patients and visitors
Administration of—appointments system
—treatment room
—clinics
Repeat prescriptions
Registrations

Telephone
Enquiries
Appointments
Advice

Filing
All patient contacts
Results and correspondence
Summaries and disease registers

Clerical
Computer registrations and recalls
Copy and audio-typing
Photocopying
Word processing

Health promotion
Appropriate use of health services
Notice-board information
Leaflet information

Housekeeping

HEALTH VISITOR

Employed by the District Health Authority and usually attached to a particular practice. Professionally independent.

They are RGNs with midwifery or obstetric experience and special training in health visiting.

Duties

Prevention of all types of ill health especially in young and old
Detection of ill health and surveillance of high risk groups
Recognition of need and mobilisation of resources
Health education
Provision of care including support in times of stress or illness
Duty is to visit all children, under 5, at least once

COMMUNITY MIDWIFE

Employed by District Health Authority usually 'group attached'. Professionally independent.

Duties
Antenatal clinic care
Antenatal classes
Intrapartum care
Postnatal care
Advice on infant feeding
Statutory duty to attend a mother for 10–28 days following delivery.

DISTRICT NURSING SISTER

Employed by District Health Authority and usually 'group attached'.

Practice in their own right and responsible for their own case-load. Sister leads a team which may include Staff nurses, SENs and Auxiliaries.

Nursing assessment of patients
Prescribe, direct and evaluate nursing care
Terminal care
Bereavement counselling
Rehabilitation towards patient independence
Health education
Liaison with other agencies
Facilitating financial and other benefits
Caring for the carers (supporting families)
Teaching
Personal development

DISPENSER

Employed by the practice

Duties
Dispensing
Recording prescriptions
Submission of prescriptions to PPA
Collecting prescription charges and payment to FHSA
Stock control and ordering
Repeat prescriptions
Cleaning returned bottles
Dispensary security

STAFF CONTRACTS

Employment law is complex and legal advice should be sought when drawing up staff contracts. The BMA can advise. The major legislation is the Employment Protection (Consolidation) Act (1978).

The contract
Name and address of employer and employee
Date of start of employment
Job title and description
Place of work
Salary and method of payment. Incremental date and review
Hours of work. Overtime. Weekends and statutory holidays
Holiday entitlement and pay
Health and safety at work
Sickness or injury—terms and conditions, sick pay benefit
Maternity leave
Pension
Rights to notice and termination of employment
Details of any fixed contract
Disciplinary rules and procedures
Grievance procedure
Social security pensions—whether contracting out certificate is in force
Method of altering contract
Statement whether previous employment counts as part of continuous employment
Responsibility for personal property
Confidentiality of information
Professional Indemnity or Insurance

STATUTORY SICK PAY

Covers all employees sick for four or more days except those specified in the booklet *Quick Guide for Employers* (NI 268) and notably those earning less than the lower weekly earnings limit for National Insurance.

Is payable for up to twenty-eight weeks thereafter sickness benefit becomes payable.

SSP is remibursed to the employer by witholding it from the monthly payments of National Insurance.

Employer must keep careful records of employee's days of absence.

Employee must complete form SC1 or employer's equivalent.

STATUTORY MATERNITY PAY

Statutory Maternity Pay (SMP) replaces maternity pay payable under previous legislation. (Refer to the Department of Social Security *Quick Guide* NI 268.) There are detailed qualifying rules and SMP is paid at two rates depending on length of service and number of hours worked per week.

HEALTH AND SAFETY AT WORK

The most important pieces of legislation are:

Health and Safety at Work Act (1974)
Offices, Shops and Railway Premises Act (1963)
Employers Liability (Compulsory Insurance) Act (1969)
Control of Substances Hazardous to Health Regulations (1988)

It is important to provide information, training and supervision to ensure health and safety at work

Issue written statement of general policy on health and safety to employees
Provide training in use of equipment
Provide standing orders and 'Policy File'
Ensure proper maintenance and safety of equipment
Keep Accident Book and Accident Report Forms, e.g. HMSO Book F2059 and Forms 2508
Ensure premises have Fire Certificate or meet approval of Fire Officer
Ensure staff Fire Training including evacuation
Display Fire Instructions
Ensure satisfactory toilet and washing facilities and supply of drinking water
Ensure satisfactory heating (16°C), lighting and ventilation. Display thermometer
There are legal requirements for floor space (40 ft^2/ employee), breathing space (400 ft^3/employee) and seating when working
Provide storage for employees' personal effects
Ensure safe storage of drugs and chemicals (Medicines Act also applies)
Assess risks to health of hazardous substances (including chemicals, fumes and micro-organisms)
Ensure control measures for hazardous substances are used
Monitor exposure of employees to hazardous substances and health surveillance as appropriate
Provide and enforce Health and Safety policy

HEALTH AND SAFETY AT WORK—
continued

Ensure safe disposal of waste, particularly clinical waste
and 'sharps'

Display notices warning of any hazards

Consider appointing a 'Safety Officer'

Obtain Employer's Liability Insurance and display
certificate

Seek advice of Crime Prevention Officer about security and
FHSA Medical advisor about security of drugs

Consider first-aid training for staff

HIRING AND FIRING STAFF

Hiring
Establish a job description
Advertise—outline of job
—qualifications required
—Reply to include:
age and sex
curriculum vitae
references
Short list applicants
Take up references
Arrange interviews
  Intelligence
  Experience
  Special skills
  Attainments
  Interests
  Circumstances, environment and family commitments
  Attitudes to confidentiality
  Ability to deal with people

Firing
Trade Union and Labour Relations Acts and Employment Protection Acts outline procedures for industrial tribunals and grounds for dismissal.
This excludes employees who:
  work less than 8 hours a week
  work less than 16 hours a week
    and employed for less than 5 years
  have worked less than 26 weeks
Grounds for dismissal
Misconduct—employee should be given a stated number of written warnings
—Act which leads to final dismissal must be severe
—Gross misconduct would not require warning
Incapability—usually requires careful comparisons
Redundancy
Other substantial reasons

120

Practice management

ALLOCATION TO A DOCTOR

A patient may apply to the FHSA to be allocated to a doctor if he has been unable to register with practices in his area. The allocation committee will allocate to a specific doctor. There is usually an understanding that the specified doctor will keep the patient registered for a reasonable time.

CHANGING DOCTOR

Doctors
To remove a patient from his medical list the doctor applies in writing to the FHSA who then inform the patient. Removal is effective 14 days after application is received.

Patients
If a patient wishes to change doctor he/she completes and signs his/her medical card and submits it to the new doctor. The requirement for the previous doctor to sign Part B has been removed under the new contract but many patients will still have old style medical cards.

REGISTRATION WITH A NEW DOCTOR

Patient completes medical card FP4 (FP1 if old card missing), FP13 if ex-services, FP58 for new babies
Complete the following forms as appropriate
   FP28A   for patients in a 'dispensing' area
   FP/CHS for Child Health Surveillance/Under 5s)
   FP1001 for contraceptive services
   FP24   for maternity services
Request completion of Health Questionnaire
Give copy of Practice Information Leaflet
Offer Health Check (letter given or sent)

FREE NHS PRESCRIPTIONS

1. Automatic entitlement to free prescriptions
Women 60 or over, men 65 or over
Under 16
Under 19 and still in full time education
Receiving Income Support or Family Credit
Partner of someone receiving Income Support or Family Credit
Pregnant or had a baby during last 12 months
War or MOD disablement pension (for prescriptions for that disability)
Suffering from one or more medical conditions
    permanent fistula requiring continuous surgical dressing or appliance
    epilepsy requiring continuous anticonvulsant therapy
    continuing physical disability preventing leaving home without help
    conditions for which specific substitution therapy is essential
        diabetes mellitus
        myxoedema (hypothyroidism)
        hypoparathyroidism
        diabetes insipidus or other forms of hypopituitarism
        Addison's disease or other forms of hypoadrenalism
        Myasthenia gravis

2. Entitlement due to low income
Those not entitled to free prescriptions and who need about 5 or more items per month should be advised to consider buying a 'season ticket' (prepayment certificate)—apply on Form FP95 (EC95 in Scotland) from Post Offices, chemists, FHSA or Social Security Offices.

Further details on form P. 11.

COMPLAINTS

Complaints against practitioners should normally be made to the FHSA within 13 weeks. Complaints against hospitals should first to be taken to the hospital administratrom the DHA or the RHA, or via the Community Health Council. Complaints may then be taken to the Health Service Commissioner who is independent and whose job it is to investigate many complaints concerned with hospitals and other health services. Complaints should normally be made within 1 year. The HSC does not investigate any matter which the complainant could have brought before a tribunal or a court of law.

TIMES OF AVAILABILITY OF DOCTORS TO PATIENTS

All GPs are required to obtain FHSA approval for the times and places at which they propose to be available to patients under the NHS.

Full-time unrestricted GPs

These GPs will normally be available for 42 weeks per year and for not less than 26 hours per week over 5 days. The 26 hours may be spread over 4 rather than 5 days when they are also undertaking health related activities elsewhere within the public service.

The hours 'available to patients' means time spent in consultation in surgery, clinics or visits and includes travelling time.

Job shares/part-time practitioners

GPs jointly available for 26 hours per week will be included in the medical list provided they practice in partnership and the aggregate of hours is not less than 26 hours per week.

Part time GPs

GPs may apply to work half-time (less than 19 but not less than 13 hours per week) or three-quarter time (less than 26 hours but not less than 19 hours).

Job sharing and part-time GPs are required to be available for 42 weeks per year but are not required to be available 5 days a week.

Associates

The new Associate Allowance allows 2 more single-handed isolated GPs jointly to employ an associate doctor.

Restricted list and services principals

Restricted list principals care for a restricted category of patients connected with a particular establishment or organisation.

Restricted services principals undertake to provide services limited to child health surveillance, contraceptive, maternity or minor surgical services.

TIMES OF AVAILABILITY—continued

Assistants
A doctor must have FHSA approval to employ an assistant(s) for more than 3 months in a 12-month period whether or not the employment qualifies for an assistant's allowance.

Doctors' retainer scheme
This scheme helps doctors under 55 years who are currently not working more than one day a week to:
1 maintain GMC registration and medical defence organisation membership;
2 attend at least 7 educational sessions a year;
3 to take a professional journal;
4 work from one-half day per month to a maximum of one full day per week.

The scheme is administered by Regional Health Authority and applications should be made via local Clinical Tutors.

ANNUAL REPORTS

Information to be provided in annual reports*

Staff
  numbers but not names
  duties and hours
  qualifications and training

Premises
  changes in last year
  changes planned

Referrals
  referrals inpatient/outpatient/self referral
  general surgery
  general medicine
  orthopaedic
  rheumatology/physical medicine
  ENT
  gynaecology
  obstetrics
  paediatrics
  ophthalmology
  psychiatry
  geriatrics
  dermatology
  neurology
  GUM
  X-ray
  pathology
  other

Outside commitments
Arrangements for comments
Drug formularies
  repeat prescriptions

*Schedule IE of DoH *Terms of Service*

PRACTICE INFORMATION LEAFLET

Information to be included in practice leaflets*

Full name, sex
GMC qualifications
Date and place of first registration
Consultation times
Appointments system (if operated)
Obtaining urgent and non-urgent appointments
Obtaining urgent and non-urgent home visits
Off duty cover
Repeat prescription system
Dispensing arrangements
Clinics
Numbers and roles of staff
Services provided—child health surveillance, minor
    surgery, maternity, contraceptive services
Single handed/partnership/partner/jobshare/group
    practice
Comments on service
Practice area
Disabled access
Assistants
Training and teaching

*Schedule ID of DoH *Terms of Service*

LOCAL DIRECTORIES

FHSAs are required to publish local directories as well as maintaining a medical list.

Name of GP
Register qualifications and date of award
Date of birth or date of first full registration
Surgery address and telephone number
Names of partners or GPs in 'Group'
Practice area (map)
Appointment system
Days and hours of attendance
Nature of frequency of clinics
Number of assistants and trainees
Number of other persons employed or available; nature of
    service and average hours worked
Terms of consent for deputising services
Whether on—obstetric list
             —child health surveillance list
             —minor surgery list
             —contraceptive service list
Whether relieved of responsibility for certain periods
Whether temporary (Reg 19 Appts)
Whether restricted list/services GP
Particular clinical interests
Languages spoken by GP and staff

AUDIT

A medical audit is a study of some part of the structure, process and outcome of medical care, carried out by those personally engaged in the activity concerned, to measure whether set objectives have been obtained and thus assess the quality of care delivered (Sheldon 1981).

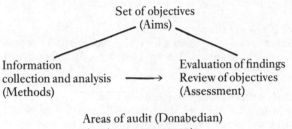

Set of objectives
(Aims)

Information collection and analysis (Methods) → Evaluation of findings Review of objectives (Assessment)

Areas of audit (Donabedian)
structure—components
process—actions
outcome —results

OVERSEAS VISITORS

Hospital services
People not ordinarily resident in the UK have to pay special statutory charges for most NHS hospital treatment unless specifically exempt. Generally 'ordinarily resident' means living lawfully in the UK voluntarily for a settled identifiable purpose and usually for more than six months.

Ambulance transport
There are no NHS charges for ambulance transport as provided to UK residents. Arrangements for repatriation should be made privately.

Family practitioner services
The hospital charges do not apply to FPS. The acceptance of a particular person, including an overseas visitor, remains at the discretion of a doctor within his conditions of service.

Overseas visitors requiring immediately necessary treatment owing to accident or emergency should be treated under the NHS (SFA para 4).

Most visitors from other EEC countries can be regarded as entitled to NHS treatment except when they have come specifically for treatment—in which case they should generally have the prior approval of their insurance institution and should be able to produce Form E112.

FPS charges (including prescription charges)
Overseas visitors are liable to the statutory charges for FPS services on the same basis as UK residents.

Domiciliary nursing
Is provided to overseas visitors on the same basis as to UK residents without additional charges.

OVERSEAS VISITORS - continued.

Reciprocal arrangements

The UK has reciprocal arrangements with the following countries for treatment of their nationals when the need for treatment arises during a visit to the UK.

Anguilla	Isle of Man
Australia	Malta
Austria	Montserrat
British Virgin Isles	New Zealand
Bulgaria	Norway
Channel Islands	Poland
Czechoslovakia	Portugal
Falkland Islands	Romania
Finland	St Helena
German Democratic Republic	Sweden
Gibraltar	Turks & Caicos Is.
Hong Kong	USSR
Hungary	Yugoslavia
Iceland	

Patients from other countries or those who have come to the UK specifically to obtain treatment without entitlement may be treated privately.

Private treatment

GPs should clearly advise patients of their entitlements under reciprocal arrangements and whether they are being treated privately or under the NHS. Patients referred to hospital should be advised to enquire at the hospital about their detailed entitlement and liabilities.

Further information

Consult FPN 353 or contact hospital or FHSA administrator.

DISPENSING PRACTICES

General practitioners may provide a dispensing service for their patients when authorised to do so. The following conditions apply:

The area must be designated as 'rural' by the FHSA

The patient must live more than a mile from a chemist

Outline consent must be obtained from the Rural Dispensing Committee set up under the 'Clothier' report. This is a central committee and applications are made through the FHSA

The patient must complete FP28A

Method of payment
The Capitation Fee System has been abolished

Drug tariff method
The basic price or 'net ingredient cost'
An on-cost allowance of the net cost
A container allowance per prescription
A dispensing fee

ORGANISING A DISPENSARY

Design and layout
Security and controlled drugs
Staff training and supervision
Tablet counters, bottles, labels
Ordering and stock control
Documentation
Claiming fees
Financial audit
Prescription charges
Collection and transport
Repeat prescriptions
Drug record in case notes
Drug audit and formulary
Relationship with pharmacists
Relationship with suppliers
Drug information service
Patient information cards

TREATMENT ROOM

Examination
Sphygmomanometer
Stethoscope and foetal
   stethoscope
Ophthalmoscope,
   auroscope, torch,
Scales
Height measure
Tape measure
Bunsen burner or spirit
   lamp

PR tray and proctoscope,
   sigmoidoscope
PV tray and specula
Patella hammer
Tuning fork
Laryngeal mirror
Nasal speculum
Vision charts
Colour vision charts
Audiometer
Fetal ultrasound

Investigation
ECG
Peak flow meter
Microscope and slides
Urine cell counting
   chamber
Haemoglobinometer
Blood Sugar Meter
Dipsticks

Centrifuge
Refrigerator
ESR equipment
Needles and syringes
Swabs
Magnifying goggles

Treatment
Suturing equipment
Dressings and bandages
Wax hook
Ear syringe
Lotion thermometer
Dressing tongs
Gloves
CO_2 snow apparatus
Various forceps
Spongeholder
Clip removers
Suture scissors
Ring cutter

Bandage scissors
Scalpel
Razor
Orange sticks
Airway
Anaesthetic equipment
Resuscitation equipment
Eye tray
Diathermy
Autoclave and steriliser
IUCD equipment
Enternox set
Oxygen set

Waste disposal
Clinical waste

Sharps

CONSULTING ROOM

Size

Combined consulting/examination room —minimum 11 m²
or consulting room   —minimum 9.5 m²
with examination room   —minimum 4.5 m²

Construction

Sound proof
Hand-washing facilities with running water
Privacy for patients
Desk and chairs
Couch and step
Modesty blanket
Heating and lighting
Shelves and storage
Telephone
Patient call system
Access for disabled

Equipment

Diagnostic and administrative (see p. 224)
Reference books
Rectal tray and proctoscope
Vaginal tray and speculae
Peak flow meter and placebo inhalers
Eye charts
Colour vision charts
Paediatric assessment equipment
Height rule
Weighing scales
Toy box
Box for notes
In/out tray
Dictation equipment
Rubber stamps and pad
Waste-paper basket and sharps box
Note pads and stationary supplies
Full range of forms

TELEPHONE ANSWERERS

Telephone answerers out of hours are often alone, are more likely to be dealing with emergencies and are less likely to have received any training.

Equipment
  Record book and check lists

Training
  Use of telephone system, bleeps, radios
  Method of answering
    Format to be used
    Manner/attitude—reassurance
                  —use of caller's name

  Information to be obtained and recorded
    Caller's name, address, telephone number and relationship to patient
    Patient's name, present location, home address (if different) age, registered GP
    Nature of problem
    Degree of urgency

  Training to deal with particular problems
    Panicking callers
    Suicidal calls
    Semiconscious callers
    Aggressive/abusive callers
    Hoax callers

Advice to be given to callers in case of
      Collapse/unconsciousness
      Difficulty in breathing
      Pregnant, labour, miscarriage
      Abdominal pain
      Fits and febrile convulsions
      Croup
      Accidents and falls
      Poisonings
      Psychiatric emergency
      Suicides

TELEPHONE ANSWERERS—continued

Procedure for doctor going on call to areas of risk
    Details of destination
    Expected time of arrival, departure and return home
    Action to be taken if failure to return
        —doctor
        —other patients

Information to be available to answerer
    Other doctors, practice bypass number
    Other sources of advice
    Practice manager
    District nurses
    Midwife
    Community psychiatric nurse
    Social services routine/emergency
    Deputising service
    Hospitals—casualty
    Police
    Undertaker
    Chemists (including out of hours rota)
    Alcoholics Anonymous
    Samaritans
    Citizens Advice Bureaux
    Ministers of religion
    Taxis
    Poisons Information Service (see p. 212)
    Major accident procedure

LOCUMS

Overall responsibility for patient care remains that of the employing doctor.

Locum must be fully registered with GMC and Medical Defence Organisation. Certificates should be shown to employing doctors.

Qualifications and experience of locum should be sufficient to bring 'a level of care and skill appropriate to GPs'. Check experience required—maternity, child health surveillance, minor surgery.

Establish requirements for accommodation and transport.

Written agreement covering
  Self employed status and contract for service
  Duration of locum, length of notice
  Payment: rate of pay, extra responsibilities of service payments, private fees
  Provision of car and payment of expenses or mileage
  Board and lodging, single or family accommodation
  Workload, rota, and extent of duties
  Night and weekend responsibilities

'Locum Folder'
  Weekly timetable
  Names of hospitals and consultants
  Lists of telephone numbers
  Practice policies and protocols
  Practice formulary
  Names and duties of nursing ancillary and attached staff
  Treatment room services
  On call and bleep arrangements

Supply of statutory claim forms, emergency drugs and equipment.

The BMA can advise on agreements, current rates of pay and employment code.

The FHSA should be informed if the locum is not a principal on the Medical List, is providing night cover or if the employing doctor is to be absent for more than a week.

ASSESSING A DEPUTISING SERVICE

Services offered
Details of contracts
Costing of services

Medical personnel
Selection procedure used
Standard of practice required
Suitable for obstetric and GP hospital duties
Adequate numbers for the population served

Supporting Staff
Experience of telephonists and drivers

Priority of calls
Effective assessment of urgency

Response to calls
A doctor should be involved in the giving of any advice

Communications
Adequate radio or telephone links with control room, the doctor, and the patient's own GP as necessary

Continuity of care
Effective reporting of all cases and the action taken to GP

Records
Full records of all telephone calls made to the deputising service

AGE-SEX REGISTER

Administration
Population profile
FHSA claims and targets
Previous registrations and 'turnover'

Screening 'call and recall'
Cytology
Blood pressure

Immunisation programmes
Rubella
Tetanus and polio
Under 5s

Disease register
Chronic diseases, e.g. hypertension, diabetes
Disabled patients
'At risk' patients
Rare clinical conditions
Overdose and self-injury patients

Geriatric serveillance

Bereavement file
Bereavement visits
Cancer register

RCGP COLOUR CODES

Colour	Group	Overprinted	Notes
Red	Hypersensitivity	HYPERS. TO	Drug sensitivities, severe toxic reactions, idiosyncrasies, major allergies
Brown	Diabetes	DIAB.	Types I and II
Yellow	Epilepsy	EPIL.	
Green	Tuberculosis	TB.	Active, arrested or cured
Blue	Hypertension	HYPERTEN.	By agreed criteria for the therapy or surveillance
White	Long term maintenance therapy	LTM THERAPY	E.g. steroids, thyroid, Vit B_{12}, antibiotics
Black	Attempted suicide		
Chequered	Measles	MEAS.	
Pink Pale yellow Light blue			For individual doctor's use

COMPUTERS IN PRIMARY CARE

Administration
Patient register
Word processor
Dispensary stock-control
Staff salaries
Finance   FHSA targets

Age–sex register

Disease register
'At risk' disease groups
Morbidity register

Prescriptions
Repeat prescription print-outs
Drug interactions

Patient recall
Preventive care
Item of service payments
Cervical cytology screening
BP screening

Patient data base
New patient questionnaires
Past medical history
Relevant family history

Research
Case finding
Controls
Self-audit

Education
Reference 'book' for medical information
Information source for teaching

Data Protection Act

BUYING A COMPUTER

Additional check list
Before buying a computer take independent advice e.g. RCGP Information Technology Manager, Primary Health Care Specialist Group of British Computer Society (0235 850389) or FHSA Computer Facilitator.

Is a computer necessary?

Does it fit your exact needs?

Can the system be expanded or adapted as your needs develop?

How many people can use it at one time?

How many functions can it perform at one time?

How good is its security?

What back up facilities are there to protect your records?

What maintenance is available and how quickly?

Is telephone advice available?

Will the supplier supply a replacement during repair?

What insurance is available?

What training is available
  on site?
    at what cost?

How good are the manuals?

Is there a user's group?

Can you see the system demonstrated?

Can you contact other customers?

Can you lease, rent or buy?
  What is included?

IN THE NOTES

Summary Card

Name	Sex
Address	Date of birth
Telephone number	Marital status
Occupation	Partner's occupation
Allergies	Height
Immunisation status	Ideal weight
Smoking	Parity
Alcohol	Contraception record
Solvent abuse	Chronic illness (colour codes)
Cytology record	Colour coding

Family history
Serial recordings of weight and blood pressure

Medical History—
in chronological order
Recurrent diseases
Persistent diseases
Severe diseases
Accidents
Fractures
Hospital admissions
Operations

Life events—
in chronological order
Births
Marriage and divorce
Deaths
Leaving home
New jobs and unemployment
Moving home
Successes and disappointments

Continuation card abbreviations

A	Attendance of patient
V	Visit to patient
C	Certificate
NV	Night visit
ET	Emergency treatment
T or P	Advice by 'phone

CERTIFICATES

MED 3	Standard statement of illness by the doctor
	To be issued after 7 days of illness
	Vague diagnosis—submit supplementary MED 6
	Not to be issued retrospectively
	Not to be issued without examination
MED 5	Special statement by the doctor
	Use when MED 3 is inappropriate
	For a previous illness if patient was seen but no certificate was issued
	For an illness verified by another doctor
MED 6	Special statement to RMO
	Explanation of a 'vague diagnosis' on MED 3
	Explanation of the true diagnosis, if not known by the patient
RM7	Referral to the RMO
	For second opinion as to whether patient is fit for work
SC1	Self certification by the patient to be completed after four days' illness
	Required for the first seven days' of illness
	Also used as the claim for for SSP, sickness benefit and invalidity benefit
CW8	Certificate of pregnancy
MAT B$_1$	Certificate of expected confinement issued after 26 weeks
	Submitted with BM4 to the DHSS by the patient
MAT B$_2$	Certificate of confinement

Northern Ireland
In Northern Ireland names of certificates differ slightly

NHS FORMS

NHS forms can be obtained from the Family Health Services
Authority by completing Form FP30A.

Completed NHS forms should be sent to the local FHSA or
to the FHSA appropriate to a patient's area if not on a practitioner's own list.

General medical
FP4   Medical Card.
FP5/6   Medical Record Envelope (male and female).
FP7/8   Continuation Card   (male and female).
FP22 A-E   Request for FHSA to return patient's notes.
           Application used when a patient has left an
           area, emigrated or died.
FP28A   Supply of Medicines and Appliances Prescribed
           by the Doctor ('Dispensing Form').
FP58   Application for inclusion on doctor's list (babies
           only).
FP69   Notice of removal of patient from doctor's list.
           To be effective within 6 months.
FP92   Prescription charge exemption certificate.
MCW01   Co-operation record card for maternity patients.
MCWO2A   Envelope for record card for maternity patients.

Treatment
FP10   Prescription Form.
FP19   Record of treatment of temporary resident. For
           patients staying in the area between 24 hours
           and 3 months.
FP31   General anaesthetics service claim form.
FP32   Emergency treatment claim form. For patients
           staying in the area for less than 24 hours.
FP81   Night visit
FP82   Application for arrest of dental haemorrhage.
FP106   Immediately necessary treatment.

NHS FORMS—Continued

Services

FP24	Maternity Medical Services. Certificate and claim for payment applicable for doctors on the obstetric list. This form is also used for emergency maternity services including treatment of miscarriage.
FP24A	Maternity Medical Services. Certificate and claim for payment applicable for doctors not on the obstetric list.
FP73	Vaccination and immunisation claim.
FP1001	Application for contraceptive services. Annual application.
FP1002	Contraceptive services – fitting of intra-uterine device.
FP1003	Contraceptive services – treatment of person temporarily absent from home.

Allowances

FP16	Application for inclusion on the Medical List. This constitutes the legal contract with the FHSA. It also includes application for maternity and contraceptive services.
FP16A	Application for filling a practice vacancy in reply to an advertised vacancy.
FP30A	Requisition by doctor for certificates, prescriptions and other claim forms from the FHSA.
FP45	Trainee Practitioner Scheme. Claim for payment to pay the trainee's allowance.
FP79	Application for seniority allowance.
FP81	Application for night visit fee.

New Contract Claim Forms

FP/CHS	Child Health Surveillance.
FP/AA	Associate Allowance.
FP/LSR	Locum Allowance for single-handed rural GPs attending courses.
FP/UMS	Undergraduate Medical Students.
FP/RF	Registration Fee (New Patients).
FP/HPC	Health Promotion Clinic.
FP/MS	Minor Surgery.
FP/TCI	Targets—Childhood Immunisation.
FP/TPB	Targets—Preschool Booster.
FP/TCC	Targets—Cervical Cytology.
FP/PEA (1)	Postgraduate Educational Allowance.
FP80	Employment of Assistant.
LOC 1	Additional Payments during sickness.
LOC 4	Additional Payments during confinement.
LOC 6	Claim for Locum payments.
PS 1,2,3 & 4	Practice Staff Scheme.

Scotland and Northern Ireland
Certain of the forms listed above have different numbers in Scotland and Northern Ireland. For precise details, contact Health Boards as forms change frequently.

NHS PAYMENTS

The system of payments for general practitioners under the National Health Service is detailed in the Statement of Fees & Allowances (The Red Book).

Basic practice allowance and additions for

Designated areas	Employment of an assistant
Seniority	Associate allowance

Standard capitation fees depending on patient's age

Payment for services

Child health surveillance	Services as anaesthetist
New patient registration (health check)	Arrest of dental haemorrhage
	Postgraduate education
Night visits	Trainee scheme
Vaccinations and immunisations	Doctor's retainer scheme
Contraceptive services	Education of undergraduate
Health promotion clinics	medical students
Maternity services	Minor surgery
Temporary residents	Rural practice
Emergency treatments	Supply of drugs and appliances

Payments for targets

Childhood immunisation	Cervical cytology
Preschool boosters	

Special arrangements for

Practitioners in inducement areas
Locums for rural single-handed GP's education
Sickness
Confinement
Prolonged study leave

Arrangements for reimbursement for

Rent and rates	Improvement grants
Practice staff	Computing costs

Arrangements for GPs

Providing limited services
With preserved nights from previous contract
With transitional payments over change in contract

TARGET PAYMENTS

On April 1 1990 Target Payments were introduced for payment for cervical cytology and immunisations for children. These payments are made quarterly at two rates depending on the level of uptake by the target population. The higher rate is three times the lower rate.

For each activity there are two sets of calculations. The first establishes whether or not a target level has been reached and the second calculates the actual payment.

Calculating the target

Target population at first day of quarter	Uptake higher payment	Required lower payment
Cervical screening Women 25–64 (21–60 in Scotland) excluding those who have had hysterectomy	80%	50%
Childhood immunisation all children aged 2	90%	70%
Preschool boosters all children aged 5	90%	70%

Calculating the payment

If a target is reached, payment will depend on the size of the practice population in the relevant target group and the proportion of the target population who received the procedure within the general practice.

HEALTH PROMOTION CLINICS

Under the new Contract fees are payable for Health Promotion Clinics.

    Initial surveillance for disease disability and health problems
    General advice and counselling on the maintenance of good
       health
    Well woman and well man clinics
    Anti-smoking
    Alcohol control
    Diet
    Exercise counselling
    Diet and stress management
    Heart disease prevention
    Diabetes
    Other areas may be allowable at FHSA discretion
        —asthma
        —hypertension
        —psychological counselling

Clinics may cover more than one area and normally must last for at least one hour and attract at least 10 patients per session.

MINOR SURGERY

GPs with appropriate training and experience may be admitted to the minor surgical list and can claim for payment for up to 60 operations per GP per year. The operations must be performed by a GP on the minor surgical list assisted, where appropriate, by a suitably trained assistant who would normally be a nurse or another doctor.

The premises, facilities and equipment must satisfy FHSA guidelines including sterilisation of equipment and tissue histology as appropriate.

Procedures qualifying for payment

Injections	—intra-articular
	—peri-articular
	—varicose veins
	—haemorrhoids
Aspirations	—joints
	—cysts
	—bursa
	—hydrocoele
Incisions	—abcesses
	—cysts
	—thrombosed piles
Excisions	—sebaceous cysts
	—lipoma
	—skin lesions for histology
	—intradermal naevi, papilloma, dermatofibroma and similar conditions
	—warts
	—ganglions
	—removal of toe nails (partial and complete)
Curette, cautery and cyocautery	—warts and verucae
	—other skin conditions e.g. molluscum contagiosum
	—ligation of varicose veins
	—removal of foreign bodies
	—nasal cautery

DEPRIVATION PAYMENTS

Deprivation payments are made for each payment resident in an area identified as 'deprived' using the Jarman Index.

Factors: Elderly living alone
Under 5s
Unskilled
Unemployed
Single-parent households
Overcrowded households
Persons who have moved house
Residents in ethnic minority households

Each factor is weighted according to impact on workload. Census data for electoral wards (England) and post code areas (Scotland) was used to derive a score (Jarman UPA 8 Score). In Wales information on standard mortality rate and housing conditions was included (Jarman WUPA Score).

Deprivation payments are made at three levels according to score.

FEES FOR SERVICES

The British Medical Association publishes details of the statutory, agreed and recommended fees for a wide variety of part-time medical services.

Services for which fees may be charged
Reports for attendance allowance
Insurance examinations and reports
Cremation certificates
Examination of drivers and pilots
Pre-employment medicals
Incapacity certificates (other than National Insurance)
Services to the Police, Coroner or Courts
Immunisation for travel abroad where a fee is not payable by
    the Family Practitioner Committee

Services for which fees may not be charged
Death and stillbirth certificates
Maternity certificates
National Insurance certificates

CERTIFICATION

Abortion before 28th week
No notification required. No certificate required.

Stillbirth
Certificate to be signed by doctor and midwife. Also Registrar must be notified by parent, guardian, or house owner within 42 days (21 days in Scotland).

Neonatal death
Certificate to be signed by registered doctor if death occurs within the first 28 days of life.

Live births
No certification but notification to the DHA by hospital, midwife or doctor within 36 hours. Also notification to Registrar by parent guardian, or house owner within 42 days.

Death
Certificate may be signed by the doctor if the deceased has been seen by him within 14 days and there is no doubt of the diagnosis.

If the deceased has not been seen within 14 days or only after the death has occurred, the Registrar must inform the Coroner.

If the diagnosis is in doubt, report the death to the Coroner who may then authorise certification. In this case the appropriate box on the reverse of the certificate should be completed.

Scotland and Northern Ireland
In Scotland and Northern Ireland the regulations may differ.

CREMATION FORMS

A   Request for cremation completed by close relative of the deceased.

B   First medical certificate completed by attendant doctor who must have seen the patient before death.

C   Confirmatory medical certificate completed by an independent doctor registered more than 5 years, having consulted the attendant doctor and examined the body.

D   Replaces forms B and C when it is completed by a pathologist following a post-mortem examination.

E   Replaces forms B and C when it is completed by the Coroner.

F   Authority to cremate. It is completed by the Medical Referee for Cremation.

RENT AND RATES

The rent and rates of practice accommodation is reimbursible by the FHSA if certain criteria are met. Full details are set out in the SFA (Red Book)

Rates, levied by local authorities or water authorities will be reimbursed.

Rent can be calculated in a number of ways.

Paid to a landlord or local authority

Notional rent for owner—occupiers

Cost rent for new separate purpose built premises or their equivalent. This is a rent related to the cost of building work rather than the current market rent.

Improvement grants
Are available towards the cost to doctors of improving existing medical practice premises and can be one-third of the cost of approved work and professional statutory fees.

Source of income
There are now many sources of loans for GP's—banks, some building societies and the GPFC—which offer loans and lease-back scheme.

Any GP considering new premises or improvements is advised to consult his FHSA.

INCOME TAX

Your accountant may require the following information to prepare your annual tax return:

Income tax return form
Form P60
Form P45
Book of accounts
Details of pensions
Pay slips
Unearned income—tax dividends
              —building societies
              —deposit accounts and income not taxed at source
              —royalties, copyright fees
Personal expenses—secretarial expenses
              —stationery and postage
              —renewals and repair of equipment
              —laundry and cleaning
              —proportion of household expenses
              —on-call telephone answering
General expenses
Travelling expenses
Motoring expenses
Life assurance and pension annuity policies
Mortgage statement
Rent received and expenses incurred
Payments under deed of covenant
Charges against income
Professional subscriptions
Medical books and equipment bought
Alimony/maintenance
Marital status
Children born during year
Dependant relatives

ACCOUNTING SYSTEMS

Discuss with your accountant a system suitable for your practice

Main account book for bank transactions
Cash book—income
Cash book—payments
Wages book
Fees ledger
Purchase invoice file
Income statements file
Receipts file
Bank and building society statements
Cheque stubs
Paying-in books

Columns in main account book

Expenditure

Date
Narrative/description
Cheque No.
Salaries—staff eligible FP reimbursement
Salaries—other staff
Partners' drawings
Light and heat
Phones and communications
Rent and rates

Insurance
Drugs and medical supplies
Stationary and printing
Locum fees
Petty cash
Cleaning and laundry
Repairs and renewals
Capital
Sundries

Income

Date
Narrative
Ref. No.
FHSA
Dispensing
Medical insurance and reports
Private patients
Outside appointments

Vocational training

DECLARATION OF GENEVA

At the time of being admitted as a Member of the Medical Profession:

I solemnly pledge myself to consecrate my life to the service of humanity;

I will give to my teachers the respect and gratitude which are their due;

I will practise my profession with conscience and dignity;

The health of my patient will be my first consideration;

I will respect the secrets which are confided in me;

I will maintain by all the means in my power the honour and the noble traditions of the medical profession;

My colleagues will be my brothers;

I will not permit considerations of religion, nationality, race, party politics or social standing to intervene between my duty and my patient;

I will maintain the utmost respect of human life from the time of conception; even under threat, I will not use my medical knowledge contrary to the laws of humanity.

I make these promises solemnly, freely and upon my honour.

HIPPOCRATIC OATH

'I swear by Apollo the Physician, by Aesculapius, by Hygieia, by Panacea, and by all the gods and goddesses, making them my witnesses, that I will carry out according to my ability and judgement, this oath and this indenture. To hold my teacher in this art equal to my own parents; to make him partner in my livelihood; when he is in need of money to share mine with him; to consider his family as my own brothers, and to teach them this art, if they want to learn it, without fee or indenture; to impart precept, oral instruction, and all other instruction to my own sons, the sons of my teacher, and to pupils who have taken the physicians' oath, but to nobody else. I will use treatment to help the sick according to my ability and judgement, but never with a view to injury and wrongdoing. Neither will I administer a poison to anybody when asked to do so, nor will I suggest such a course. Similarly I will not give to a woman a pessary to cause abortion. But I will keep pure and holy both my life and my art. I will not use the knife, not even, verily, on sufferers from stone, but I will give place to such as are craftsmen therein. Into whatsoever houses I enter, I will enter to help the sick, and I will abstain from all intentional wrongdoing and harm, especially from abusing the bodies of man or woman, bound or free. And whatsoever I shall see or hear in the course of my profession, as well as outside my profession in my intercourse with men, if it be what should not be published abroad, I will never divulge, holding such things to be holy secrets. Now if I carry out this oath, and break it not, may I gain forever reputation among all men for my life and for my art; but if I transgress it and forswear myself, may the opposite befall me.'

ROYAL COLLEGE OF GENERAL PRACTITIONERS
(14 Princes Gate, London SW7 IPU)

Aims
To encourage, foster and maintain the highest standards in general practice.

Membership
Full membership by pass in MRCGP examination
Associate membership available to those who have not taken or are ineligible to take the examination.
The MRCGP examination is held twice a year and consists of written papers and oral examinations.

Eligibility
Fully registered for at least four years, of which two have been in general practice or completion of a vocation training course or approved equivalent

Benefits
Membership constitutes the only postgraduate qualification in primary care in the UK
Quality initiative— Fostering good general practice
Accommodation and facilities for functions
Faculties organise a range of functions, meetings and conferences throughout the country
Electronic technology department—computers
Press Office—deals with the media
International affairs
Working parties have been set up involving many topics
College library—a major reference library
Information service—information on physical and organisational aspects of practice. Publishes record cards for sale
Online search—computerised services to researchers
Prestel
Publications—journal, occasional papers, booklets, and RCGP Members Reference Book
Education—courses, examinations and educational research
Research—research units and projects
Information technology—computers

162

PRIORITY OBJECTIVES

Patient care

Problem definition
Recognise common physical, psychological and social problems
Assess patients beliefs, effects on daily living, effect on psychological state, patient's expectations of the doctor
Understand the principles of problem definition
Cope with own anxieties

Management
Chose with the patient appropriate management
Involve other members of the team
Use records effectively
Prescribe appropriately
Manage life events and crises
Provide appropriate care and support
Make appropriate referrals
Involve and educate the patient
Be aware of the cost

Emergency care
Diagnose and initially manage all acute emergencies

Prevention
Understand the principles of case finding, health education and screening
Understand systems for information handling
Provide effective preventive services

Communication

Patients
Consultants tasks (see p. 165)

Partners, team and other professionals
Understand the roles of other professionals
Understand meetings
Understand others' needs
Use personal resources appropriately

PRIORITY OBJECTIVES – Continued

Organisation

The practice
Manage the practice effectively
Monitor practice activity
Solve problems appropriately
Understand the NHS contract and regulations
Understand legal and financial aspects of practice
Use appropriate technology
Manage change and innovation

Personal organisation
Manage time
Delegate appropriately

Community
Respond to the community's health needs
Participate in community affairs

Professional values
Be aware of personal values
Recognise social, cultural and organisational factors that affect work
Maintain ethical principles
Respond to others with tolerance, respect and flexibility
Submit to critical peer-review
Maintain physical and mental health
Balance personal and professional commitments
Accept appropriate responsibility

Personal and professional growth

Identify personal strengths and weakness
Recognise changing needs in others
Define own educational needs
Adapt to change
Be aware of personal limiting factors

Printed by permission of the Oxford Region Course Organisers and Regional Advisers Group from occasional paper No. 30 (RCGP), 'Priority Objectives for General Practice Vocational Training'.

STUDYING THE CONSULTATION

Increasing importance is being given to the study of the consultation during vocational training. The use of video recording is an accepted part of this. There are many models of consultation proposed and maps and rating scales to use.

Models of consultation
Consultation Tasks (Pendleton, Schofield, Tate & Havelock: *The Consultation, An approach to Learning and Teaching*, Oxford University Press)

1 To find out why the patient came
   (a) nature and history of problems
   (b) aetiology
   (c) patients ideas, concerns and expectations
   (d) effects of problems
2 To consider other problems
   (a) continuing problems
   (b) at risk factors
3 With the patient, to choose an appropriate action for each problem
4 To achieve an appropriate shared understanding of the problem with the patient
5 To involve the patient in the management and to encourage him or her to accept an appropriate degree of responsibility.
6 To use time and resources appropriately
   (a) in the consultation
   (b) long term
7 To establish or maintain a relationship with the patient which helps to achieve the other tasks

STUDYING THE CONSULTATION—
continued

Stott & Davis: The Potential in each Primary Care Consultation (*J. Royal Coll. Gen. Pr.* 1979, **27** 201–5)

A	B
Management of presenting problems	Modification of help seeking behaviour
C	D
Management of continuing problems	Opportunistic health promotion

Byrne & Long: *Doctors Talking to Patients*, HMSO 1976

1 The doctor establishes a relationship with the patient
2 The doctor either attempts to discover or actually discovers the reason for the patient's attendance
3 The doctor conducts a verbal or physical examination or both
4 The doctor, or the doctor and the patient, or the patient (in that order of probability) answer the condition
5 The doctor, and occasionally the patient, detail the treatment or further investigation
6 The consultation is terminated normally by the doctor

Learning and Teaching (*Future General Practitioner—learning and teaching*, RCGO 1972)

Problem presented	Solution proposed
Problem examined	Solution examined
Problem defined	Solution implemented

Pereira Gray: *Training for General Practice*, 1982 Macdonald & Evans, Plymouth

Problem presented	Solution presented
Problem discussed and defused	Solution discussed and defined
Problem agreed with doctor	Solution agreed with patient

RULES FOR DISCUSSING VIDEO CONSULTATIONS ('PENDLETON RULES')

1 Briefly clarify any matters of fact
2 The doctor on the video goes first and must discuss first what he did *well*.
'What did you do well?'
3 Observers then discuss what he did *well*.
What did he do well?'
4 The doctor on the video then describes what he did not do well *and* recommendations for change.
'How would you have done it better?'
5 Observers then discuss what he did not do well *and* recommendations for change.
'How could he have done it better?'

VOCATIONAL TRAINING REQUIREMENTS*

Vocational training requirements
Before becoming a principal in general practice, a period of training of four or more years is required from the date of provisional registration. This comprises the equivalent of twelve months in a NHS general practice as a trainee and a minimum of three years in hospital posts in NHS hospitals or with HM forces. At least one year of the hospital posts must include two or more of the following specialties:

General medicine
Chest medicine
Traumatic surgery or accident and/or emergency work
Obstetrics and gynaecology
Paediatrics
Psychiatry
Geriatrics
Otorhinolaryngology
Dermatology
Ophthalmology
Anaesthesia

An alternative is a special course arranged by or with a university including experience in hospitals and general practice.

The doctor must hold a certificate of prescribed or equivalent experience.

Full information may be found in the NHS Statement of Fees and Allowances.

* Information from 'The Statement of Fees and Allowances payable to General Medical Practitioners' by permission of the Department of Health and Social Security.

SELECTING A VOCATIONAL TRAINING SCHEME

Seek the advice of the Regional Adviser, the local course organiser and past and present trainees on the scheme.

Organisation
Sequence and duration of job rotation
Flexibility in jobs offered
Compatability with previous experience
Attitudes to women and part-timers
Attitudes to change after starting course or early cessation
Contact with GP trainers whilst in hospital jobs
Feedback and trainee participation in organisation
Opportunity to visit prior to selection
The Contract

Hospital jobs
Experience and training offered and relevance to GP
Duties, rotas, on-call arrangements
Opportunities for further diplomas and degrees
Time off for GP or other teaching
Accommodation offered

GP
Characteristics of training practices (see p. 174)
Facilities offered to trainee
Characteristics of trainers and their partners
Location of practices and travelling involved
Travel and telephone arrangements

Teaching
Organisation of time and subjects
Training methods and attitudes
Attitudes to additional study leave or courses
Library and reference facilities

CURRICULUM VITAE

Name	Qualifications
Address	Age
Telephone No.	Marital status
School	Scholarships and prizes
University	Degrees, distinctions and prizes
Postgraduate experience	Hospital jobs
	Diplomas and degrees
	Publications and research
	Other appointments
	General practice experience

Medical interests
Career interests
Medical societies and communities
Other interests

GMC registration number
Defence Society membership
Certificate of prescribed or equivalent experience
Name and address of referees

Accompanying letter
Nationality
Religion
Health
Family details
Availability

THE TRAINEE CONTRACT

The trainee should agree on terms of service with the trainer. This may take the form of a contract or letter of employment which should include at least the following:

Dates of commencement and duration of contract
Notice required for termination of contract
An undertaking by the trainer to teach and advise
Salary and frequency of payment as in 'Statement of Fees and Allowances'
Leave: holiday, illness, maternity and study leave
Medical equipment to be provided by trainer
Provision of car or car allowance
Membership of a Defence Organisation
Full registration with GMC
Working hours, night and weekend duties
Accommodation—if applicable
Settlement of disputes by arbitration

The terms of the contract should be subject to Terms of Service for Doctors (as set out in NHS General Medical Services) and the Employment Protection Acts.

The BMA and Defence Societies have produced model contracts for trainees and assistants joining practices.

PAYMENT OF TRAINEES

The trainee undertaking hospital jobs is paid by the Health Authority as any other junior hospital doctor under NHS General Whitley Council conditions of service. When undertaking the trainee year in general practice, the trainee is employed by his trainer. He is not self employed. The trainer must not pay the trainee any salary or emolument in excess of the amounts specified in the SFA.

The trainee pays the relevant employee's portion of the National Insurance and Superannuation. This is usually deducted at source.

The Employment Protection & Safety at Work legislation applies to trainees.

The SFA should be consulted as it details:

Rates of trainee salary, weightings and increments

Allowances for motoring expenses

Reimbursement of telephone installation charges

Reimbursement of removal, house purchase, storage and other expenses

Reimbursement of travelling expenses and subsistence involved in obtaining accommodation

Reimbursement of losses arising from educational arrangements for children

Allowances during searches for accommodation

Reimbursement of miscellaneous expenses on moving

Allowances for continuing commitments relating to previous accommodation

Payment of rent of unoccupied property

Payment of expenses when on call

Payment of excess rent

Payment of interview expenses for traineeships

Payments during sickness. During sickness lasting less than two weeks the trainee is usually paid by the trainer less SSP deductions and this should not affect recognition of training. For longer than this, consult FHSA

Maternity leave

Examinations: travelling expenses and subsistence is reimbursable but *not* the examination fees

Payment of subscription to professional defence organisation

EDUCATIONAL EXPENSES AND SUBSISTANCE

Trainees

Under Section 63 of the Health Services and Public Health Act (1968) expenses and subsistence allowance are claimable by trainees attending postgraduate meetings and courses approved by Postgraduate Deans. Trainees must obtain approval before attending courses outside their own regions. The rate of reimbursement increases periodically. Claim forms are issued whilst attending the course and signature of the attendance register is mandatory. The limit on claims per year varies from region to region.

In Wales—Section 2; in Scotland and Northern Ireland the forms are different.

Principals

Section 63 has been abolished for GP principals. The new Postgraduate Education Allowance covers these expenses. Qualification for the allowance involves 25 days (or equivalent sessions) on courses on approved subjects spread over a 5 year period. There are special transitional arrangements in 1990 and 1991 and on entry to general practice.

Approved subject areas
1 Health promotion and prevention of illness.
2 Disease management.
3 Service management.
Approval is given by Regional Advisors or Postgraduate Deans.
Courses can be periods of formal education (e.g. at a Postgraduate Education Centre) or informal (at a surgery). A course may run continuously for a prescribed period or consist of separate sessions. Distance learning packages may also be accredited.

SELECTING A PRACTICE

The practice organisation
List size and characteristics
Appointments system
On-call work
Workload
Work share
Annual, sick, maternity and study leave
Telephone cover
Age, sex and disease registers
Record systems
Research
Teaching
Outside interests
The primary health care team

The practice facilities
Premises: health centre, surgeries, ownership
Treatment room
Dispensary
Equipment
Computer
Library
Teaching aids

The partners
Ages and sexes, of partners
Medical interests and qualifications
Ethical and moral issues
Decision making
Partners' motivation
Attitudes to innovation
Attitudes to the incoming partner
Priorities claimed for seniority
Outside interests
Spouses and families
Politics and religion

SELECTING A PRACTICE—Continued

Finance
Time to parity
Method of payment to parity
Distribution of income
NHS and private income
Inspect accounts
Tax liability
Cost of joining practice
Future expenses

The practice area
Local hospitals
Consultants
Waiting lists
Liaison with other practices
Laboratories and paramedical services
Postgraduate education
Local medical politics

The community
Housing
Transport
Shops
Schools
Cultural and leisure facilities
Proposed building and development
Local politics

FORMS ON ENTRY TO PRACTICE

The forms required on entry to practice will vary between FHSAs. Always consult the FHSA Administrator at the earliest opportunity.

Applicants for single-handed vacancies must apply on the forms specified by the FHSA—FP16A.

Applicants for vacancies in partnerships should apply as advertised.

All successful candidates should check that FHSA and Medical Practices Committee approval is complete before entering any commitments—particularly financial.

FORMS TO BE COMPLETED
(where appropriate)

Application for inclusion on medical list	(FP16)
Application for addition to basic practice allowance for vocational training	(FP78)
Application for NHS superannuation scheme	(SS14(RD))
Declaration of partnership	(FPC pro forma)
Declaration of time spent in GP (for BPA)	(FPC pro forma)
Authorisation of voluntary levy for local medical committee	(FPC pro forma)
Authorisation for rural dispensing compensation fund	(FPC pro forma)
Authorisation to banks for crediting NHS remuneration by FHSA	(FPC pro forma)
Application for inclusion in obstetric list	(FPC pro forma)
Application for designated area allowance	(FP76)
Application for seniority allowance	(FP79)
Application for initial practice allowance	(FPC pro forma)
Application for inclusion—child health surveillance	(FPC pro forma)
—minor surgery	(FPC pro forma)
Application for postgraduate education allowance	(FP/PEA)

DOCUMENTATION ON ENTRY TO PRACTICE (as appropriate)

GMC—certificate of full registration (current)

Defence Society—certificate of membership (current)

Birth certificate

Certificate of prescribed or equivalent experience issued by JCPTGP (14 Princes Gate, London SW7) or statement of grounds of exemption (with supporting evidence)

National Insurance number

P45 or statement of tax position

Certificate of training in family planning (JCC)

Evidence of postgraduate obstetric qualification or experience or previous inclusion in an FHSA Obstetric List as detailed in application form for inclusion in obstetric list

Evidence of receipt of seniority payments/date first inclusion in a medical list

Evidence of experience—child health surveillance
                    —minor surgery

Intended place of residence (consult FHSA before financial commitment)

THE PARTNERSHIP CONTRACT

Partnership contracts are complex and a solicitor's advice should be sought. LMC secretaries should be contacted for details of GMSC checklist—voluntary monitoring scheme.

The following topics should be covered as appropriate:

Who is to form the partnership

*Properly executed and witnessed

Commencement date and duration of contract

*Arrangements and grounds for termination of contract/dissolution of partnership

*Details of practice promises and equipment, ownership, valuation, incoming/outgoing partners

*Terms of rental or purchase

*Division of income and expenditure—private and NHS

*Practice profits, shares, percentages and arrangements to pool. Guaranteed share—option to convert to profit sharing

*Each partner to receive annual accounts

*Profit share not tied to list size

Financial responsibility for personal and partnership expenses, debts and tax, shares of assets and gifts

*Definition of income to go to practice or partner (including seniority payments and PGEA)

Superannuation arrangements

*Arrangements for signing cheques

*Named practice banker and accountant

Restrictions on private residency and distance from surgery

Restrictions on other business or medical commitments

Membership of defence organisation and medical register

Terms of employment of staff

Arrangements concerning communications and telephones

*Retirement and expulsion of partner

Selection of a new partner

Length and priority of holiday and study leave etc.

Arrangements about representation/outside appointments

Engagement of locums

Arrangements in case of military service

*Allowable absences, annual extra leave, maternity/paternity leave, compassionate leave, study leave, sabbaticals

THE PARTNERSHIP CONTRACT—continued

*Patients' rights to register with doctor of choice
*Arrangements on death or chronic illness of partner, sickness
  insurance, sick leave
Personal debts not to be secured against partnership assets
Any restrictive clauses to be made clear
*Settlement of disputes by arbitration

*Covered in GMSC monitoring of partnership agreements check list.

Emergency care

ACUTE LEFT VENTRICULAR FAILURE

Assessment

Previous history
Hypertension
Myocardial infarction
Valvular heart disease
Paroxysmal cardiac arrhythmia
Orthopnea

Circulatory state
Pallor
Cyanosis
Shock
BP
Pulse
Heart murmurs
Triple rhythm
Signs of right heart failure

Respiratory state
Bilateral basal crepitations
Pleural effusions
Frothy blood-stained sputum

ACUTE LEFT VENTRICULAR FAILURE—
continued

Action

Frusemide 40–80 mg IV (further 40 mg if no response in
   2 hours)
Diamorphine 5 mg IV or IM (add prochlorperazine 12.5 mg
   IM if necessary)
Oxygen
   Aminophylline 250–500 mg IV slowly if no response to
   above treatment or if asthma cannot be excluded
Nurse patient sitting up

Referral
   Failure to respond to therapy
   Poor home circumstances
   Suspected pulmonary embolism
   Persistent arrhythmia

ASTHMA

Assessment
Previous history
Precipitating factors
    Allergy
    Stress
    Exercise
    Infection
    Environment
Current medication
Cyanosis and pallor
Pulse
BP
Signs of heart failure
Drowsiness
Expiratory wheeze
Hyperinflation
Peak flow assessment and respiratory rate

ASTHMA—continued

Action
Salbutamol
  Nebulised respirator fluid.
  'Nebule':
    adult 2.5–10 mg 6 hourly
    child 2.5–5 mg 6 hourly
  Intravenous:
    adult 2.5 mg
  Intramuscular:
    adult 5 mg
    child 8 μg/kg
  (Alternatives are terbutiline, adrenalin or aminophylline)
Hydrocortisone 100–200 mg, IV or IM (of paramount
  importance in acute asthma)

Aminophylline (if it is difficult to differentiate between asthma
  and acute LVF) 250–500 mg slowly IV in an adult, 5 mg/kg
  in a child

Monitor peak expiratory flow (PEF) before and after treatment

Referral to hospital:
  pulse > 120/min
  PEF < 100L/min
  no response to treatment after 30 min
  persisting cyanosis

ANAPHYLACTIC SHOCK

Assessment

Airway
Stridor
Bronchospasm
Rhinitis

Circulation
Hypotension
Arrhythmia
Tachycardia

Skin
Angioneurotic oedema
Urticaria
Rash

Gut
Abdominal pain
Vomiting
Diarrhoea

History
Allergy and exposure to allergens

Common allergens

Antibiotics	Snake bites
Anti-inflammatory drugs	Insect bites and stings
Anti-arrhythmic drugs	Various plants and pollens
Iron preparations	Nuts
Blood products	Eggs
Vaccinations	Milk
Desensitizing allergens	Shellfish

ANAPHYLACTIC SHOCK—continued

Action

Parenteral drugs
Adrenalin (1:1000) 0.5 ml s.c. (repeated at 15 minute intervals
  if necessary)

Drugs
Hydrocortisone 100–200 mg IV
Chlorpheniramine 10 mg slowly IV

Circulatory collapse
Establish IV line with electrolyte solution or plasma expander

Respiratory collapse
Maintain airway and ventilation
Oxygen
Consider tracheostomy to relieve laryngeal obstruction

BACK INJURY
Suspect spinal injury until proved otherwise.

Assessment
Circumstances of the injury
Other injuries
Clinical signs
Conscious patient
may localize pain along the spine
sphincter control
check distribution of pain for anaesthetic
check the effect of cough impulse
observe movement of limbs and digits on request
inspect reflexes and digits

Conscious or unconscious patient
palpate vertebral column
observe response to sensory stimuli—in *all* dermatomes
facilities for moving and transporting patient

BACK INJURY—continued

Action

Fractured vertebrae
Apply a cervical collar on suspicion of spinal injury
Avoid patient slumping forward or changing position
Adequate analgesia
  e.g. Entonox
  morphine 5 mg IV (with Prochlorperazine 12.5 mg)
Move patient only when necessary
  in a fully supported position
  by a planned procedure
  gently
  with all available help
Transport in a supine position with padding to lumbar and
  cervical spine, and legs padded and bound
Accompany patient during transport especially if unconscious
  and supine

Acute back strain or prolapsed intervertebral disc
Supportive position e.g. supine on firm mattress
Adequate analgesia
Muscle relaxants e.g. Diazepam 5 mg 8 hourly
Embrocation or warmth
Refer to hospital if signs of nerve compression are present

BONE INJURY

Assessment
Circumstances of the injury
Which bones are affected
Other injuries and/or shock
Signs of a fracture
    immobility or non-use (particularly in children)
    pain and tenderness
    deformity or shortening of the limb
    instability
    swelling
    crepitus
Vascular or neurological complications
Predisposing factors e.g. osteoporosis or bony metastasis
Obvious and potential blood loss

BONE INJURY—continued

Action
Establish IV line
N saline up to 1 litre to maintain BP above 100 mm Hg
  systolic
Haemacel 500 ml in 30 minutes
Immobilise the affected limb
  strap to adjacent limb
  inflatable splints
  Thomas splint or variant
Ensure adequate analgesia
  e.g. IV morphine 5 mg (with Prochlorperazine 12.5 mg)
  Entonox
  Or oral analgesics as appropriate
Consider management of other injuries
Arrange referral for
  X-ray
  Reduction of dislocation (and subsequent radiography)
  Fitting of longer term support

Potential blood loss from fractured bones

Chest wall (closed injury)	2 litres
Pelvis (closed injury)	2 litres
Femur	1.5 litres
Arm bones	1 litre
Other leg bones	1 litre

BURNS

Assessment
Circumstances of burns
Distribution and extent of burns

'Rule of nines'

head	9%
trunk-front	2×9%
trunk-back	2×9%
upper limb	9%
lower limb	2×9%

Depth of burn—erythema or anaesthesia
Associated shock
Airway and respiratory involvement
Other injuries

BURNS—continued

Action
Cool with water
   extinguishes the fire
   reduces pain
   reduces severity
   dilutes chemical burns
Resuscitate if necessary
i.v. fluids or plasma expander if available
Oxygen
Adequate analgesia
Leave blisters intact
Cover with sterile dressings

Home care
Small superficial burns
Cover with antiseptic dressings e.g. Flamazine for 10 days—
   change when necessary

Hospital care
Extensive burns—7% baby
            —10% child
            —15% adult
Burns to face, hands and perineum
Explosion injury or airway involvement
Large full thickness burns requiring skin grafting
Delayed healing of superficial burns

CARDIAC ARREST

Assessment

A-B-C of resuscitation
Assess
    Surroundings and continuing danger
    Patient consciousness
    Assistants and helpers
    Brief history from any witnesses
Breathe
    Look for chest movements
    Listen for breath sounds
    Feel for expired air
Circulate
    Look for cyanosis, pupil reaction and spontaneous movement
    Listen to the heart
    Feel for carotid or femoral pulse

CARDIAC ARREST—continued

Action—unassisted

Airway
Extend the neck
Remove foreign bodies, false teeth, secretions and vomit

Mouth to mouth ventilation
Extend neck
Pinch nose
Lips sealed over patient's lips
Breathe out till chest rises
Allow exhalation
2 quick breaths
Feel for carotid pulse
    pulse present: ventilate 12–16/minute
    pulse absent: CardioPulmonary Resuscitation (CPR)

Chest compression (CPR)
Heel of one hand 3 cm above xyphisternum
Second hand on top
Arms straight and vertical
Depress sternum 4–5 cm
Compression rate 80/min 15 times then ventilate twice and
    repeat the sequence

Call for support

CARDIAC ARREST—continued

Action—with full support
Continue CPR
Secure airway with endotracheal tube
Give oxygen
Establish ECG monitor

Asystole
Defibrillate 200J then 200J then 360J
then Adrenaline 1 mg IV
then Atropine 2 mg IV

Ventricular fibrillation
Defibrillate 200J then 200J then 360J
then adrenaline 1 mg IV
then defibrillate 360J
then lignocaine 100 mg IV
then defibrillate 360J then 360J and repeat

QRS complex but no pulse
Adrenaline 1 mg IV
Consider calcium chloride 10 ml of 10% solution

Every 5 minutes give adrenaline 1 mg IV
Consider sodium bicarbonate 50 ml of 8.4% solution
Transfer to hospital

CROUP (LARYNGEAL STRIDOR)

Assessment
Onset of symptoms
Inspiratory stridor
Barking cough
History of inhaled foreign body
Fever, pallor, cyanosis
Pulse (tachycardia)
Respiratory rate
Respiratory effort (intercostal recession, use of accessory
   muscles)
Distress and level of consciousness
Avoid inspection of throat if epiglottitis is suspected

Other causes of stridor

Laryngotracheobronchitis	Laryngeal oedema
Epiglottitis	Diphtheria
Inhaled foreign body	Whooping cough
Laryngeal trauma	

Action

Home care
For simple laryngitis sit the child up in a humid, steamy
   atmosphere
Consider antibiotics (amoxycillin as first choice)
Advise warm drinks
If condition settles quickly (within 30 min) reassess later

Referral to hospital
No relief with initial management
Increasing respiratory distress or cyanosis
Inadequate social circumstances
Suspicion of epiglottitis, inhaled foreign body, laryngeal trauma
   or oedema, or diphtheria

CHEST INJURY

Penetrating wounds and crush injuries, with or without 'flail-segments', are clinically obvious and require urgent action.

Blunt injury in the early stage is not clinically obvious but this too requires urgent action.

Assessment
Circumstances of the injury
Associated injuries
Airway and degree of respiratory distress
Inspect skin changes
    central and peripheral cyanosis
    chest wall
    deformity of ribs or sternum
    paradoxical movement
    penetrating wounds
    surgical emphysema
Trachea and mediastum—deviation from centre
Auscultatory changes
Signs of internal haemorrhage
    chest capacity: 2 litres
    abdomen capacity: 2 litres
Aortic injury
Oesophageal injury
Diaphragmatic injury

CHEST INJURY—continued

Action
Close any open chest wound
Maintain the airway
Ventilate if necessary
Arrange urgent transfer to hospital
Insert intercostal tube (with or without flutter valve) into second
    intercostal space anteriorly when a tension pneumothorax is
    present.

COMA

Assessment

Respiration
Establish that the airway is not obstructed
Note rate and rhythm of breathing

Circulation
Assess adequacy of pulse rate and rhythm; BP

Level of consciousness
Record the time of examination and the
   eye opening
   best verbal response
   best motor response

Other signs
Colour, hydration, skin changes
Evidence of injury—bleeding and fractures
Incontinence
Ketones or alcohol on breath
Pupils, fundi and reflexes
Neck stiffness
Rectal temperature
Evidence of overdose (drugs, vomit)

Witness report
Onset and duration of coma
History of injury
Patient's medical and drug history
Social circumstances

Differential diagnosis of coma

Cerebral	Respiratory failure
epilepsy	biochemical imbalance (Na, Ca, PO$_2$,
stroke	CO$_2$, pH)
trauma	hepatic failure
infection	hypothermia
Metabolic	Addison's disease
diabetes	uraemia
hypoglycaemia	**Toxic**
Circulatory	alcohol
low cardiac output (all causes)	overdoses

COMA—continued

Action

Resuscitate—Assess, Breathe, Circulate
Insert IV drip and endotracheal intubation if possible
Control bleeding
Exclude spinal injury and major fractures
Do not move the casualty unnecessarily
Recovery position—in the absence of intubation consider
  nursing the casualty in the three-quarters prone position
Try to establish diagnosis for further emergency treatment
Organize transport to hospital

Glasgow coma scale

Eyes open	Best verbal response	Best motor response
Spontaneously	Orientated	Obey commands
To speech	Confused	Localises pain
To pain	Inappropriate	Flexion to pain
None	Incomprehensible	Extension to pain
	None	

CONVULSION

Assessment
Detailed description of convulsion—from a witness
Onset, duration sequence of events and subsequent symptoms
    or signs
Medical history
    Fever
    Recent head injury
    Epilepsy
    Diabetes
    Withdrawal of alcohol or drugs
Respiratory rate
Pulse
BP (sitting and standing)
Signs of injury
    Incontinence
    Fever
    Focus of infection
    Raised intracranial pressure (meningism)
    Neurological deficit

Causes of convulsions
Febrile convulsion
Hypoglycaemia (in neonates or diabetes)
Hypocalcaemia (in neonates)
Epilepsy
Tumour
Stroke
Syncope
Hyperventilation

CONVULSION—continued

Action

Telephone advice
Cool a febrile child
Lay in three-quarter prone position

First aid
Maintain airway
Remove dentures
Three-quarter prone position
Avoid aggressive management
Reassure attendants

Anticonvulsants
Diazepam 5–10 mg IV or p.r. (0.2 mg/kg BW) repeat if
    necessary in adults
Paraldehyde 5 ml IM (0.1 ml/kg BW) repeat in opposite leg
    in adults if necessary

Brown paper bag in **hyperventilation**
Glucogen IM or IV 1 mg ⎫ (**hypoglycaemia** in adults
Dextrose 50% IV 20 ml ⎭ with diabetes)

Referral
Immediate referral of neonates
Persistent convulsion (> 15 mins)
Incomplete recovery in 3 hours (to exclude meningitis)
Age < 1 year or > 75 years (for investigation of epilepsy)
Second febrile convulsion for investigation and prophylactic
    anticonvulsants
Signs of raised intracranial pressure

ECLAMPSIA

Assessment
Confirm diagnosis
Patient must be
    pregnant
    hypertensive
    convulsing
Obstetric history
Epileptic history
BP
Neurological examination
Fundal height
Foetal heart rate

Action
Control convulsion
Diazepam 5 mg IV (repeat if necessary)
Control BP
Diamorphine 5 mg IV (repeat if necessary)
Consult with obstetric flying squad
Continue to monitor
    pulse
    pupils
    BP
    reflexes
    conscious level
    foetal heart rate

ELECTROCUTION

Assessment
Establish circumstances of the electrocution
    voltage, amps and duration of current
    the source of the current
    the points of entry and exit from the body
Do not approach patient until it has been confirmed that there is
    no continuing risk
Check:
Airway and respiration
Cardiovascular status
Level of consciousness and response
Extent of burns
Associated injuries
Involvement of internal structures and organs

Action
Eliminate the source of electrocution
Ensure personal safety
Ventilate and/or resuscitate as necessary
Treat shock
Treat burns
Transfer to hospital

HEAD INJURY

Assessment
Check airway and respiration
Establish circumstances of the injury
Check for other injuries
Level of consciousness
    Eye opening
    Best verbal response
    Best motor response
CNS examination particularly
    Pupil response and size
    Fundi
Check for
    CSF leakage from nose or ears
    Skull fracture
If conscious assess the degree of pre- and post-traumatic
    amnesia

HEAD INJURY—continued

Action
Maintain airway if comatose
Organise transfer to hospital if there is
    Loss of consciousness
    Significant pre- or post-traumatic amnesia
    Skull fracture
Monitor
    Pulse
    BP
    Respiratory rate
    Pupil response
    Limb movements
    Level of consciousness e.g. Glasgow coma scale

Glasgow coma scale

Eyes open	Best verbal response	Best motor response
Spontaneously	Orientated	Obey commands
To speech	Confused	Localises pain
To pain	Inappropriate	Flexion to pain
None	Incomprehensible	Extension to pain
	None	

HYPERGLYCAEMIA

Assessment
Known diabetic with
    inadequate control
    intercurrent infection
Undiagnosed diabetes

History
Malaise
Weight loss
Infection
Thirst
Frequency of micturition
Abdominal pain

Signs
Gradual onset
Flushed
Bounding pulse
Ketotic breath
Dehydration
Vomiting
Confusion
Coma

Urinalysis positive for glucose (+/− ketones)
Blood sugar > 20 mmol/litre

Action
Blood sample for glucose, creatinine and electrolytes
Soluble insulin 10 units s.c. or i.m.
IV fluids if dehydrated: normal saline 500 ml in 30 min
Organise immediate transfer to hospital

HYPOGLYCAEMIA

Assessment
Known diabetic on insulin or oral agents

History
Excessive dosage
Excessive exercise
Delayed meals
Rapid onset of symptoms

Symptoms
Dizziness
Sweating
Hunger
Fainting
Nausea
Palpitations
Paraesthesia
Headache

Signs
Irrational or aggressive behaviour
Cold and clammy
Tachycardia
Coma
Incoordination
Pallor
Hypotension
Convulsions

Urinalysis negative to glucose
Blood sugar < 2.5 mmol/l

Action
Blood sugar for glucose
Conscious patient
   Oral glucose or carbohydrate enriched meal
Unconscious patient
   Glucagon 1 mg IM
   Dextrose 50% 20 ml IV (repeat if necessary)
Urgent referral if no response
Review medication and diet

HYPOTHERMIA

Assessment
Rectal temperature less than 35°C after 5 min with low reading
  thermometer
Cardiovascular state (particularly arrhythmia or bradycardia)
Level of consciousness
History of
  injury
  dementia
  drug abuse
  exposure
  hypothyroidism
  social problems

Action
Resuscitation
  Attempt even after prolonged cardiac arrest
Refer to hospital
  rectal temperature less than 32°C
  home care inappropriate
  coma
  arrhythmia
  CCF
  stroke
  impaired respiration
  head injury
  overdose
Home care
  rectal temperature more than 32°C
  room temperature 25–28°C
  adequate supervision.

OVERDOSE AND SELF-INJURY

Assessment
Circumstances of the event from patient or witnesses
    Time and place
    Sequence of events
    Details of implements used
    Quantity and nature of drugs used
    Evidence of overdose
    Evidence of alcohol abuse
    Degree of suicidal intent
    Involvement of others
General enquiry
    Previous attempts
    Recent mental state
    Medical history
    Psychiatric history
    Social and environmental factors

Examination
Present mental state
Level of consciousness
Examination of injuries
General examination
Brief inspection of the house for alcohol, drugs or toxic
    chemicals

Action
General supportive measures
Collect remaining drugs, containers, or implements
Contact poison centre (see p. 212)
Arrange transport to hospital
Arrange care for dependents

PAEDIATRIC RESUSCITATION

The effective care of children in an emergency requires confidence and precision. The chart opposite offers guidance for such care. The notes below offer guidance in the use of the chart.

The graph represents age plotted against weight for the 50th centile boy-girl average.

To the left are shown dimensions of endotracheal tubes, which correlate well with age.

Below is a table showing various drug doses for use in cardio-respiratory arrest or other urgent conditions.

Also included are defibrillator settings and suggestions for initial fluid infusion in hypovolaemia.

The doses comply with the present Resuscitation Council guidelines.

If the weight is already known drug dosage may be estimated by moving directly downwards from the weight axis.

If age but not weight is known dosage may be estimated by tracing across the graph and then down to the dose.

If neither is known a rapid stretched out length may be measured with a tape measure and the non-linear scale above the graph used to estimate drug dosage.

From: Oakley PA. Inaccuracy and delay in decision making in paediatric resuscitation, and a proposed reference chart to reduce error. *Br. Med J.* 1988; **297**: 1 October.

Based on the guidelines of the Resuscitation Council (UK).

PAEDIATRIC RESUSCITATION—continued

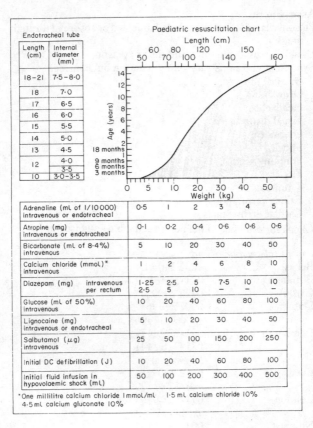

	18–21	7·5–8·0

Endotracheal tube

Length (cm)	Internal diameter (mm)
18–21	7·5–8·0
18	7·0
17	6·5
16	6·0
15	5·5
14	5·0
13	4·5
12	4·0
	3·5
10	3·0–3·5

Paediatric resuscitation chart

Adrenaline (mL of 1/10 000) intravenous or endotracheal	0·5	1	2	3	4	5
Atropine (mg) intravenous or endotracheal	0·1	0·2	0·4	0·6	0·6	0·6
Bicarbonate (mL of 8·4%) intravenous	5	10	20	30	40	50
Calcium chloride (mmol)* intravenous	1	2	4	6	8	10
Diazepam (mg) intravenous per rectum	1·25 2·5	2·5 5	5 10	7·5 –	10 –	10 –
Glucose (mL of 50%) intravenous	10	20	40	60	80	100
Lignocaine (mg) intravenous or endotracheal	5	10	20	30	40	50
Salbutamol (μg) intravenous	25	50	100	150	200	250
Initial DC defibrillation (J)	10	20	40	60	80	100
Initial fluid infusion in hypovolaemic shock (mL)	50	100	200	300	400	500

*One millilitre calcium chloride 1 mmol/mL   1·5 mL calcium chloride 10%
4·5 mL calcium gluconate 10%

POISONING

Assessment
Poisons may be ingested, inhaled, injected or absorbed through the skin
Establish nature, quantity and time of poison
Symptoms and signs vary with the poison but consider
    Nausea
    Drowsiness
    Headaches
    Visual disturbance
    Dyspnoea
    Shock
    Vomiting
    Fits
    Tinnitus
    Failing respiration
    Cardiac arrhythmias
Check for evidence of deliberate self-poisoning (see p. 209)

Poisons Information Services

Belfast	0232 240503
Birmingham	021-554 3801
Cardiff	0222 709901
Dublin	0001 379964
	or 0001 379966
Edinburgh	031-229 2477
	031-228 2441
	(Viewdata)
Leeds	0532 430715
	or 0532 432799
London	071-635 9191
	or 071-955 5095
Newcastle	091-232 5131

POISONING—continued

Action
Refer all cases if in doubt

Ingested poisons
Consider inducing vomiting with ipecacuanha mixture 15 ml
with a glass of water
Do *not* induce vomiting if the patient has swallowed caustic
chemicals or hydrocarbons or if the patient is comatose
Dilute the ingested poison with water or milk to drink if the
chemical is caustic or a hydrocarbon

Inhaled poison
Remove the patient from poisonous atmosphere as soon as
possible
Clear the airway

Transcutaneous absorption
Remove contaminated clothing with care
Wash the patient down

General
Monitor pulse and respiration
Resuscitate as necessary
Nurse comatose patients in the recovery position
Establish an IV line in shocked patients
Treat fits with intravenous Diazepam (5–10 mg)
Try to send sample of poison or vomit to the hospital with the
patient

PSYCHIATRIC EMERGENCIES

Assessment
Degree of social disturbance, embarrassment or threat to safety
    of self or others
History from witnesses
    Onset and progress of disturbance
    Preceding events
    Previous psychiatric history
    Drugs and alcohol

Examination
Pulse
BP
Temperature
Respiratory rate
Thyroid status
Focus of infection
Signs of trauma or intoxication
CNS signs

Mental state
Clouding of consciousness
Orientation
Concentration
Restlessness
Paranoia
Fear
Mood—euphoria or depression
Memory
Attention span
Irritability
Psychotic thoughts
Panic

PSYCHIATRIC EMERGENCIES—continued

Action
Telephone advice as appropriate
Consider need for police or ambulance assistance
Reassure patient and family or attendants
Treat any underlying condition at home or in hospital
    Diazepam 10–30 mg oral, IM, IV
    Chlorpromazine 25–50 mg oral (initially), 50–150 mg IM
    Chlormethiazole 1.5–2 gm oral or IV
    Haloperidol 30 mg oral or IM 10 mg initially in elderly or
       patients with liver or heart disease
    Propranolol 10–20 mg 6 hourly (in addition to Diazepam for
       acute anxiety)
    Brown paper bag for hyperventilation
Discuss voluntary admission to hospital with patient and
psychiatrist
Implementation of Mental Health Act 1983
'Persuasion before coercion'

ROAD TRAFFIC ACCIDENT
Ensure personal safety and wear reflective jacket
Park safely to
  protect casualties
  provide light
  warn other traffic
Co-operate with rescue services
Estimate the number and relative severity of casualties
Give clear instructions for any equipment or assistance
  required
Record relevant information and attach to patient

Assessment
Airway
Respiration
Circulation
Level of consciousness
Nature, degree and situation of injuries
Confirm or exclude spinal injuries

Action
Resuscitate
Maintain the airway
Stop any bleeding
Establish an IV line—N. saline or plasma expander
Ensure adequate analgesia
  Entonox
  Pethidine 100–200 mg IV
  Buprenorphine 300–600 μg IV slowly
Splint all suspected fractures
Avoid hypothermia
Monitor
  level of consciousness
  pupils and reflexes
  BP
  pulse

SUDDEN UNEXPECTED DEATH

Assessment
Confirm death has occurred

Establish circumstances from witness if possible

Confirm identity of deceased

Establish medical history from relatives or medical records if available

If unnatural death is suspected do not disturb the body or local environment until the police have been informed (see p. 92)

Examine the body completely unclothed and particularly check for bruising, injury and wounds.

Check the environment for evidence of possible suicide.

Action
Issue a certificate if the cause of death is known and the patient has received medical care in the last 14 days

Notify coroner's officer if a coroner's case (see p. 90)

Sympathetic support for the family in their bereavement

If the death is not reported to the coroner explain to the relatives the procedure for registering the death and offer the names of local undertakers

If there are no relatives arrange with an undertaker for the removal of the body

Arrange a post-mortem if it would help to confirm the cause of death

SHOCK

Assessment
Airway
Respiratory rate
Skin colour
Level of consciousness
Restlessness
Stridor or bronchospasm
Pulse
BP
Temperature

History
Trauma or bleeding
Chest pains
Abdominal pain
Vomit or diarrhoea
Allergen contact

Signs
External bleeding
Internal bleeding
Bone injury
Crush injury
Burns

Causes of shock
Anaphylactic shock
Blood loss (external or internal)
Cardiogenic shock
Electrolyte loss (e.g. dehydration)
Plasma loss (e.g. burns)
Septic shock

SHOCK—continued

Action
Maintain airway
Keep patient horizontal with legs elevated
Give oxygen 30% 20 l/min
Monitor
  pulse
  BP
  respiratory rate
  skin colour
  level of consciousness

Fluid loss
Stop bleeding where possible
Take blood sample for cross matching
IV line N. Saline 1 litre (sufficient to maintain a BP of 100 systolic)
Haemacel 500 ml in 15–30 min

Cardiogenic shock
IV line 5% dextrose by slow inflow
Diuretic for CCF e.g. Frusemide 50–100 mg IV
Antiarrhythmic drugs for arrhythmia
Adequate analgesia

Splint any fractured bones
Ensure adequate analgesia, e.g. IV Morphine 5 mg (repeat after 15 min)
  Entonox (avoid in chest injuries)
Avoid hypothermia
Transfer to hospital without delay
Reassure patient and family

SUDDEN LOSS OF VISION

Assessment
Onset and degree of visual loss
Preceding visual symptoms or associated symptoms (e.g. pain)
Exact circumstances of any injury
Medication
Medical history
    Visual acuity
    Visual fields
    Cornea and conjunctiva
    Retina, fundus and macula

Causes of sudden blindness

Amaurosis fugax	Central retinal vein occlusion
Migraine	Vitreous haemorrhage
Glaucoma	Retinal detachment
Keratitis	Retrobulbar neuritis
Iritis	Giant cell cranial arteritis
Central retinal artery occlusion	Trauma including foreign body

Action
Refer for ophthalmological assessment

EYE INJURY

Assessment
Exact circumstances of injury
Associated symptom (especially diplopia)
History of bleeding disorder
Inspect cornea and conjunctiva (even when lids are closed by
    haematoma)
Inspect skin and eyelids
Examine visual acuity
Examine extra ocular muscle function to assess site and size of
    injury
Avoid applying pressure to an injured globe

Causes of eye injury
Periorbital haematoma
Blunt injury
    'Blow out fracture' of orbit
Rupture of globe
    Hyphaema
    Vitreous haemorrhage
    Detached retina
    Choroid rupture
    Abrasions
    Foreign body
Perforating injury
Burns
    Toxic
    Thermal

Action
Irrigate eye with water after exposure to *toxic material*
Remove any *foreign body* under lid or in the cornea
1% Amethocaine drops and eye pad for *foreign body*
Chloramphenicol drops or ointment for *abrasions*
Referral—all other cases for hospital assessment
    Nil by mouth in anticipation of general anaesthetic

VAGINAL BLEEDING IN PREGNANCY

Assessment
Blood loss
   rate and estimated volume
   fresh or altered
   noted products of conception
Associated pain before or after onset of bleeding
Progress in pregnancy
Obstetric history
Associated symptoms
BP and pulse
Abdominal tenderness
Shoulder tip pain
Fluid in abdomen
Fundal height
Foetal movements and heart rate
P.V. state of cervix and adnexae. *Avoid* after 26 weeks of
   pregnancy

Differential diagnosis

Ectopic	Placenta praevia
Abortion	APH
Abruptio placentae	PPH

VAGINAL BLEEDING IN PREGNANCY—
continued

Action

Before 12 weeks
Reassurance and home management with *bed rest* if bleeding is
    minor and no associated pain.
Otherwise arrange *transfer* to hospital.
If shocked—clear products from cervical os IV fluid replacement

12–26 weeks
For painless minor bleed arrange early antenatal assessment for
    ultrasound scan and cardiotochogram
Urgent admission for major bleed or associated uterine pain
If shocked consider IV fluid replacement

After 26 weeks
Avoid pelvic examination
Consider placenta praevia
Consult with obstetric flying squad
Monitor foetal heart rate
If shocked consider IV fluid replacement

After delivery
Major bleed > 500 ml
Contact obstetric flying squad
IV line
Ergometrine 500 μg IV
Catheterise bladder
Bimanual compression of uterus

Consulting room bookshelf

Abortion Law, Medical Protection Society
ABPI Data Sheet Compendium, Datapharm Publications Ltd, 12 Whitehall London SW1A 2DU
British National Formulary (BNF), British Medical Association and the Pharmaceutical Society of Great Britain
The Casualty Officer's Handbook (Ellis, M.), Butterworth
Childrens' Developmental Progress (Sheridan, M.D.), National Federation for Educational Research
A Colour Atlas of Dermatology (Levene, G.M. & Calman, C.D.), Wolfe Medical
Drug Tarrif (DHSS), HMSO
First Aid Manual, St John Ambulance Association/St Andrew's Ambulance Association/British Red Cross Society
A Guide to Social Services, Family Welfare Association
Handbook of Contraceptive Practice (DHSS), HMSO
Handbook of Medical Ethics, British Medical Association
The Health Directory, Macdonald, Bedford Square Press
Immunisation against Infectious Disease (DHSS), HMSO
Legal Aspects of Medical Practice (Knight, B.), Churchill Livingstone
List of Fees, British Medical Association
Local Hospital referral list for consultants and specialities
Local Laboratory and X-ray Guidelines and Normal Values
Medical Aspects of Fitness to Drive, Medical Commission on Accident Prevention
Medical Emergencies & Treatment (Robinson, R.O.), Wm. Heinemann
Medical Evidence for Social Security and Statutory Sick Pay Purposes (DHSS), HMSO
MIMS, Medical Publications Ltd
MIMS Colour Index, Medical Publications Ltd
Notes on Clinical Side Room Methods (Medical Education Committee). Churchill Livingstone

Ocular Emergencies (Richards, A.B.), Smith & Nephew
  Pharmaceuticals Ltd
OTC Index, Medical Publications Ltd
Paediatric Vade Mecum (Wood, B.S.B.), Lloyd-Luke
Patient's Rights (National Consumer Council), HMSO
A Practical Guide to Mental Health Law (Gostin, L.),
  MIND
Practice Policies and Formulary
Pulse Blue Book: Forms and Fees (Bowles, D.), Morgan-
  Grampian
**Statement of Fees and Allowances Payable to General
  Medical Practitioners in England and Wales** (The Red
  Book), DHSS (Welsh Office), National Health Service,
  General Medical Services, HMSO
Travel vaccination chart, *Doctor* or *Pulse* publications
Using the Laboratory (DHSS), HMSO
Which Benefit?, (DHSS), HMSO

Telephone numbers

Alcoholics Anonymous ....

Ambulance ....

BMA ....

Chemists ....

Chiropodist ....

Citizens Advice Bureau ....

Community Physician ....

Coroner ....

Defence Society ....

Dentists ....

DHSS Local Office ....

District Health Authority ....

District Nurse ....

Education Welfare Officer ....

Family and Child Guidance ....

Family Practitioner Committee ....

GMC ....

Health Visitors ....

Home Help Co-ordinator ....

Hospitals ....

Marriage Guidance..

Meals on Wheels..

Midwives..

Nursing Officer..

Occupational Therapist ....

Partners..

Physiotherapists ....

Police ....

Poisons Information Service..

Probation Service..

Red Cross ....

RCGP..

RSPCA..

Samaritans ....

Social Workers..

Social Worker Emergency No...

Surgeries/Health Centres..

Taxis..

Undertakers ....

VD Clinic..

Voluntary Agencies ....

Index